Person-Centred Practice at the Difficult Edge

Edited by Peter Pearce
and Lisbeth Sommerbeck

PCCS Books
Monmouth

First published 2014

PCCS Books Ltd
Wyastone Business Park
Wyastone Leys
Monmouth
NP25 3SR
UK
Tel +44 (0)1600 891 509
www.pccs-books.co.uk

Person-Centred Practice at the Difficult Edge

A CIP catalogue record for this book is available from the British Library

ISBN 978 1 906254 69 8

Cover designed in the UK by Old Dog Graphics
Printed in the UK by Biddles Books Ltd, King's Lynn, Norfolk

Contents

Acknowledgements

The editors are grateful to PCCS Books for permission to reprint as Chapter 6 an amended version of Sommerbeck, L (2007) In and out of contact: Therapy with people in the 'grey-zone'. In P Sanders (Ed) *The Contact Work Primer* (pp. 49–60), and for permission to reprint as Chapter 12 an amended version of Sommerbeck, L (2005) An evaluation of research, concepts and experiences pertaining to the universality of CCT and its application in psychiatric settings. In S Joseph & R Worsley (Eds) *Person-Centred Psychopathology* (pp. 317–36).

The editors would also like to thank Taylor & Francis for permission to reprint Dekeyser, M, Prouty, G, & Elliott, R (2008) Pre-Therapy process and outcome: A review of research instruments and findings. *Person-Centered & Experiential Psychotherapies,* 7(2), 37–55, as Chapter 15 of this book.

Preface

The initial idea for this textbook arose from a workshop series at Metanoia Institute in London, UK, which focused on Therapeutic Practice at the Difficult Edge. These workshops explored the settings, clients and issues which have been regarded as 'beyond therapeutic reach', where many psychological therapies reach their edge and have been thought to provide little or no benefit. Such client groups have included those who are severely withdrawn, or whose ability to be in contact may be impaired due to learning disabilities or autism, psychoses, catatonic depression, trauma, dementia, terminal illness or brain damage. In fact, for some modalities, membership alone of some of the client groups represented in this text has been sufficient in itself to be an exclusionary criterion for access to psychotherapeutic engagement. The Metanoia workshop series brought together many of the authors represented here, and focused on providing a forum for participants to explore the possibility of therapeutic practice in such 'difficult edge' settings. Similarly this book aims to describe, in concrete ways, the developments of theory, practice and research with these client groups and contexts, in order to support counsellors, psychotherapists and other helping professionals to broaden the range of clients they are equipped therapeutically to companion.

The chapters provide a rationale and method for working with pre-relational and pre-expressive functioning and open up access for people usually labelled 'not for psychotherapy'. The approaches described provide a more humane alternative for supporting people who present with such difficulties – not a vague ideology, but a concrete, practical and pragmatic body of work. Contributors to this text are an international collection of therapists who, instead of taking uncomfortable experiences as markers of exclusionary criteria, have been willing to engage in the struggle to find a way of being with their clients', and their own, distress, and to look at the 'edge' where a client's world meets their own. Such edges can be defining, pivotal places of relationship – liminal spaces where two worlds clash, yet bridges can be built and change become possible.

At these times, therapist limits are frequently challenged and this can be regarded as one way of defining the term 'the difficult edge'. Difficulty is, of course, in the eye of the beholder, and for the therapist this can be when they arrive at the edge of their experience or the limit of their capacity. However, this capacity can be broadened and thus the edge moved. We hope that this book helps to demonstrate that such edges can be moved considerably by therapeutic practice which is person-centred and incorporates the invaluable example and well-established wisdom of Pre-Therapy. Defining and understanding such edges can also help to give shape and perspective to helping professions as a whole. We hope this book will prove to be rewarding and relevant, not only for therapists considering working at such edges but also for those working in more traditional psychotherapy and community settings with 'less distant' clients by providing the opportunity to deepen their understanding of the relationship they create with their clients.

Perhaps arising from its inclusive and egalitarian ethos, practitioners of the person-centred approach may have felt relatively more 'unhappy' with the idea of anybone being labelled as being 'beyond psychotherapeutic reach' than practitioners from some other models of therapy. This has, at least, been the case for both of us, and finding it possible, with person-centred therapy and Pre-Therapy, actually to reach such clients has been a joyful experience. In editing the book we have found that not only our own chapters, but also those of the other authors – even if describing difficult work and much struggle – are suffused with this joy of reaching the so-called unreachable and we hope this is communicated to readers.

Our aim was to edit a book with a distinctive focus on practice, so the first section of the book comprises by far the largest section. It is hoped that readers will also find the more theoretical and research-based material of the second and third parts of the book as helpful and supportive for their practice as we have. We are pleased to have been involved in this important, internationally collaborative project and have been humbled by the generous and inspirational offerings from contributors. We hope that it will help readers feel better equipped to reach out, and be companions to, those previously seen as unreachable. We see the chapters here as testimony to the fact that any notion of clients being beyond psychotherapeutic reach is obsolete.

Peter Pearce
Lisbeth Sommerbeck
May 2014

Part 1
Practice

Understanding posttraumatic stress and facilitating posttraumatic growth 1

David Murphy and Stephen Joseph

Introduction

Trauma has become a term that is used to describe a wide range of life events. Such events include war, genocide, torture, acts of terrorism through to natural disasters: earthquakes, tsunamis or floods. Traumatic events can also be those that occur on a more regular basis such as road traffic or industrial accidents, or interpersonal violence, rape or sexual assault through to bullying at school or work, bereavement or divorce. Yet while such events serve as a trigger, not everyone reacts in the same way. What causes one person and not another to experience adverse psychological reactions has been the subject of much theoretical work over the past few decades. This chapter is about person-centred therapy (PCT) in relation to the processing of trauma-related information. Although we use the term 'person-centred therapy', our practice is based on the principled non-directive approach founded on unconditional acceptance communicated through empathic response (Rogers, 1951). Briefly put, our unconditional positive regard and empathic understanding are emergent from, embodied within and conveyed through the expression of congruent empathic responses to the client's experience. First, we provide some background on posttraumatic stress, moving on to introduce Denise; a case vignette that will illustrate how practice relates to theory. Second, we will use the case of Denise to provide a deeper conceptualisation of trauma from within the growth paradigm of PCT, and finally, show how PCT provides a radical ontology for understanding how psychological trauma can be the springboard for transformational changes in a person's life – referred to as posttraumatic growth.

Posttraumatic stress

Whilst it is relatively common for a person to experience a traumatic event at some point across their lifespan, individual responses can vary considerably. Recent estimates suggest that by age 75 years the projected lifetime risk of developing posttraumatic stress disorder (PTSD) is only 8.7 per cent. PTSD is defined in the *Diagnostic and Statistical Manual of Mental Disorders 5th edition* (*DSM-5*), published in 2013, as consisting of four clusters of symptoms. First, the event is re-experienced through intrusive recollections. This can come through thoughts, emotions, dreams or even nightmares about what has happened. Often re-experiencing is accompanied by highly distressing affective states and in extreme circumstances the person feels as though the event is happening right there and then. Second, there are avoidance phenomena, when people try to ward off or evade being reminded of what has happened. Psychological avoidance might involve avoiding thinking about, talking about or experiencing feelings associated with the event. Behavioural avoidance might mean avoiding going to places or doing things that trigger memories of the events. Engaging in either psychological or behavioural avoidance can mean people appear to be coping with the traumatic event, yet after prolonged use, avoidance can have significant problematic consequences. Third, there are altered states of cognition or problems of emotional numbing. Fourth, there are states of heightened arousal. When the above-mentioned experiences significantly interfere with social and occupational functioning, a diagnosis of PTSD may be made.

The 12-month prevalence rate for PTSD in the US amongst adults is as low as 3.5 per cent and this is estimated to be even lower in Europe, Asia, African and Latin American countries (APA, 2013, p. 276). In a recent study looking into the length of time from an index[1] traumatic event and access to a specialist service, it was found that the average time of waiting was 15 years (Brabbins, Regel, Joseph & Murphy, 2013). Whilst at first glance this might sound a negative consequence of poor availability of services, it is important to remember that a number of those people would have been operating and functioning in life for a significant amount of that time. Also, when an individual finally reaches the psychotherapy room, our experience is that a client will often report more than one traumatic event in their lives. Both of these points highlight the resilience and resourcefulness of people following trauma.

Part of our work as psychologists over the last five years has been with trauma survivors in the specialist trauma centre where we have been committed to PCT. Maintaining a focus on PCT has been challenging, not least because statutory health services have been squeezed with regard to the range of therapies they are commissioned to provide. The squeeze on services is a direct consequence of the development and over-reliance on treatment guidelines. Notwithstanding the increase in treatment guidelines and the related commissioning policy, there has been a rise in the availability of PCT in specialist trauma services in the UK between 2007 and 2012 (Murphy, Archard, Regel & Joseph, 2013). One of the reasons for the increased availability of PCT in specialist services

---

1. An *index* event refers to what is thought to be the main traumatic event that has led to attending the clinic.

is due to the complexity and severity of trauma in the clients that we see. As a specialist tertiary service many of the clients we see have often 'been through the system' several times. Over a period of many years they have been offered a standardised approach to therapy that focused on addressing their symptoms and consequently missed them as a person. Instead of inquiring into the person's perception of what had happened to them which caused them to require therapy, these approaches focus on correcting what is believed to be not working within them. This is in no means a critique of our colleagues in therapy roles following more standardised methods; they too feel squeezed and constrained. Yet we have found it frustrating that when the therapies 'that work', according to treatment guidelines, haven't 'worked' – it is the specialist trauma service that becomes the final resource. The therapy practised in our service is typically PCT, tailored to client needs, but this is in no way recognised by funders, policy makers or guideline developers.

We find the work with trauma survivors to be interesting, personally growthful and educative. Our clients have frequently become very distressed and disturbed by the events in their lives and yet we see they are resourceful, resilient and striving towards different ways of being – we aim to help them in the person-centred way. We don't have goals for our clients but we do have a goal for ourselves, that is, to experience unconditional positive regard for the client which we communicate through our congruent empathic reflection focused on their experiencing and intended communication (Grant, 2010). To illustrate, we turn now to the case of Denise.[2]

Denise was a 40-year-old woman with two children. She entered therapy after being referred by a charitable organisation that helped survivors of domestic violence. She was experiencing considerable symptoms of PTSD.

Denise had lived in terror and subjugation for several years – during her time in the marriage she had been in a state of constant fear and hospitalised for two periods of psychotic breakdown. She also feared asking social services for help in case they removed her children. She was physically, sexually and psychologically abused in the relationship; the abuse having a sadistic element to it on several occasions. Denise feared for her life. The final decision to leave her husband John came while she was giving birth to her youngest child when her husband sexually abused her during labour while the midwife was absent from the room. This, for Denise, was the most severely degrading event in a long history of abuse, leaving her feeling utterly powerless and was the trigger that led her to finally leave her marriage taking her children, including her son Nick, who at the time of therapy was 8 years old. The focus of the therapy was on the manifold traumatic events that had occurred in her life. The following extract is taken from session 2:

---

2. All names and details have been changed and the stories of several clients have been amalgamated into the story of Denise.

Client: I'm really struggling today … [long pause], just before I was going to come out Nick started kicking off; like going absolutely off on one, I didn't know if I was even going to come today, I just thought 'what good will it do anyway?', but then I thought I've just got to give myself the chance, have a go, do something to get out of this hole that I'm in.

Therapist: Ah, like it was nearly too much to come today, Nick kicking off and the thought of this not doing any good anyway, and then there's needing to do something to get out the hole you're in right now.

Cl: Yes, more like just so desperate for some help, anywhere from anyone. I'm just so exhausted with everything … [pause] … desperate sounds so awful, I hate that feeling of being desperate, I'm so weak … so scared too …

Th: Scared too …?

Cl: Mmmm, yeah, huh, I don't know; when Nick goes off on one like that it just reminds me of, of, well you know, when I was with him [husband]. When I see him being like that it reminds me of how he used to go so crazy and I didn't know if that would be it this time …

Th: I see, so it's like when Nick goes off on one it brings back those memories of being back with your husband, and those really frightening experiences where you didn't know if he was going to kill you?

Cl: Yeah, I mean I feel like I'm right back there sometimes, like he's gonna walk right through the door and I'm not going to be able to do anything. I'm back in the corner of the room, sitting on the floor and just holding my hands on my head to cover up. I'm shaking and crying and then the kids come in the kitchen and are like, 'Mum, what you doing, what's the matter?' And then I'm like what, what, what's happened, and I can't remember what's happened, and then I remember that Nick was kicking off about the ice cream for pudding and that's how it all started. We had a row and then he goes off upstairs kicking things about on his way and then he's shouting at me and then I'm in the corner. But he's only 8 … what's wrong with me. I can't even have a row with my own 8-year-old without crumbling on the floor, I'm a wreck, a mess, so I had to come, to get some help, to try and change all this …

This extract demonstrates how the traumatic events from the past are reactivated for Denise. An argument with her 8-year-old son over some ice cream for tea provoked a response in her that took her back to a past event involving domestic abuse. Her son's behaviour was the trigger, as he 'kicked things' as he stormed to his room – this activated the trauma memory. Denise's response was to find a way to protect herself as she perceived the threat. Her emotional reaction was of fear, squatting down in a corner to try to protect herself. Nevertheless, she expressed her determination to come to therapy despite feeling helpless. The therapist is trying to reflect empathically the expressions and meanings that Denise makes of her experiences. He does not try to cajole or direct the conversation and is in no way following an agenda to expose Denise to feared stimuli – he trusts her as the one who knows where to go with the narrative as it unfolds. This kind of therapeutic dialogue continued for several sessions as Denise gradually exposed herself to her feelings in the safety of the therapy room.

It is possible to understand Denise's experiences from within the PTSD framework. For example, her son's behaviour acts as a trigger to re-experiencing symptoms. She indicates intrusive recollections of events from her past abuse experiences and accompanying these are emotional reactions that leave her feeling agitated and fearful for her life. However, as part of our work within the trauma service, it is also necessary to conceptualise her reactions from the perspective of PCT in order to provide the rationale for working with her in this way. In the vignette above, the therapist is recognising both the traumatic distress and the determination to come to therapy. Unconditionally responding to all parts of the client's experiencing is an important feature of the work and enabled Denise to feel accepted and understood as she continued to explore and make meaning of her process.

Person-centred conceptualisation and posttraumatic growth

The phenomenon of posttraumatic stress can be understood from within person-centred theory (Rogers, 1959). This has been extensively discussed elsewhere by Stephen Joseph (2003, 2004, 2005). In brief, psychological trauma refers to when people are exposed to a significant event(s) that causes a breakdown or disorganisation in the self-structure. A traumatic breakdown or disorganisation occurs when the traumatic event presents the self with an overwhelming amount of information that needs to be processed.[3] Traumatic events provide new information about the self and the world that challenges existing expectations, values and beliefs. So challenging is the conflicting information that the self-structure is placed under significant threat. It is not always possible for the new trauma-related information to be processed at the time of the trauma. Often the sense of threat is subceived as the person continues their attempts at processing after the event. When this processing becomes blocked, thwarted or is incomplete, difficulties arise that require help and support in order that the individual regains some sense of equilibrium. Thus what often makes an event traumatic is the perception, for that individual, that their integrity, either physical or psychological, is placed under extreme threat. One way in which a sense of extreme threat is experienced is when trauma-related information is in direct conflict with their existing self-structure. The new information just won't 'fit in' with the existing schema. As such, the task for trauma survivors is to move towards greater congruence between the experiences of the organism with experience of self-concept, as becomes evident with Denise in a later session:

---

3. We use the term 'process' to indicate that the traumatic experience has yet to be incorporated adaptively via assimilation and accommodation.

Session 8

Cl: So I've been thinking a lot about what's been happening at home with Nick and his storming around the house and my reactions, and I'm getting to see a bit more about what's happening to me and I don't know what to do right now about it ...

Th: OK, mmm, so, sounds like you're thinking a lot about things and feel a little confused by what you can do about this.

Cl: Yeah, it feels sort of weird as I feel a bit helpless still but maybe a bit less helpless than before, so something feels like it's helping. I mean I still get the thoughts and images flashing through my head, like one minute I'm cooking tea, that's when it used to happen or often, at tea time, he'd [husband] just go mental and start whacking me or going on and on picking at me and calling me names and then put the dinner straight in the bin or just chuck it on the floor and make me clean it up. Sometimes he even made me eat my dinner with the dog out the back ...

Th: Ah, like the helpless feeling is still there and still the memories come back, about those times when he really degraded you, belittled you and you felt really helpless right then.

Cl: I feel so ashamed, that I didn't say no, or stop him, or walk out or do something, but I had the kids to think of and I had to stay for them. I knew I wouldn't ever leave them and I had to protect them. And I think that's why I get so upset when Nick goes off on one now ... like I'm thinking 'don't you know what I went through for you?' or like 'if you knew what happened you wouldn't do this to me' and then I feel bad, I feel guilty about thinking like that ... 'cause of course he doesn't know, he was only a baby and not even born when it started.

Th: Like you think about what else you could have done and then how you stayed to protect the children, you kind of wish they knew, or maybe that someone knew about what you'd been through ...

Cl: Yeah, I mean someone to just say you did the right thing, you did your best, you couldn't have done any more than that, just someone to tell me that I did good and then when Nick goes off on one maybe I could stand up a bit more and not crumble to the floor and think I'm no good, look what I've done, look what a mess I created, I'm just totally useless ...

Th: Like if only someone would be there with you, and let you know you did the best you could; someone to be right by your side when you really need them ...

Cl: It's just so hard to know for myself, did I do enough, should I have gone earlier, what if I'd told the nurse at the hospital, told the police or told someone before I left, would it be different now? Just all these confusing questions and I just want someone to say it's alright, I did OK.

Th: So lots of questions about the things you did or didn't do, leaving you feeling like did I do enough and ...

Cl: Yeah, it's like I know really that I need to answer that for myself, I know if I could just tell myself that what I did was OK, if I could just accept myself then I'd feel better about this and if, like when he does, Nick kicks off again I'd be stronger, I'd be able to stand up and stand my ground and say 'no, it's fruit for pudding tonight' or something like that.

Th: Giving yourself some acceptance feels like it would be really good for you and help a lot in those situations with Nick where you want to stand your ground more.

Cl: Yeah, like I want to be able to feel OK about me not standing up to John and for standing up to Nick [pauses] … and I guess I want to feel OK too about not standing up to Nick. I know I have been through a lot of things, maybe I did OK to just survive that, to get through any way I could. There were times I thought the only way out was to end it all, I feel bad about that now and glad I didn't. I guess thinking and talking about it all here now with you makes me realise that I have been to hell and back three times over. Perhaps I did do OK, to just survive that.

In the section above Denise reflects on several experiences and the accompanying feelings of shame and guilt at her responses both at the time and also currently in her relationship with her son. These are painful recollections and leave Denise feeling helpless, yet there remains a dim sense of hope, a sense of carrying forward from where she is and into new areas of reflection and exposure to the trauma from the past. She expresses a need for someone to offer her an affirmation of doing the right thing. This is a dilemma for client-centred therapists as they have to decide about whether this risks reinforcing conditions of worth. The therapist's response to this is to recognise the feeling of needing something and in offering this he is conveying his empathy and unconditionality as later Denise also recognises her need to accept all of the parts of herself. As Denise internalises the therapist's unconditional positive regard and extends this to herself she is able to feel some hope for the future. Her unconditional positive self-regard enables her to see more of the totality of her experience, the enormity of the traumatic events and she feels accepting of herself in more of her reactions to it. In this way Denise is able to process her experiences, find greater congruence between what has happened to her and her self-structure.

As the person's self-structure becomes more congruent with the new trauma-related information, posttraumatic growth arises (see Joseph & Linley, 2005, 2006 for a discussion on PCT and posttraumatic growth). Posttraumatic growth refers to ways in which the struggle with trauma can ultimately be transformational in the ways in which people relate to themselves, others and to the world. Often, this is through changes in self-perception, shifts in priorities and values, or through a deepening of intimacy and meaning in relationships (Joseph, 2011). In this way, the experience of PCT leads not only to a reduction in PTSD symptoms but also to the facilitation of posttraumatic growth.

At no point is the therapist trying to make Denise do anything specific. In PCT with trauma survivors, the therapist's task is to create the environment that is conducive to growth; to experience unconditional positive regard and to communicate this through empathic reflections and statements that are the result of following the client's moment-by-moment experiencing. This approach to therapy places PCT in the position of being a radical ontology for trauma. PCT is based on the notion that the human organism is always active. Rogers (1959) referred to the human organism as having a single motive and termed this the actualising tendency. Rogers' proposal was that under the right kinds of social-environmental conditions the human organism would act in a socially constructive manner and move towards greater integration. As such, he proposed that we can have a basic trust in the human being to know, under the right social-environmental conditions, what direction to move, and in the case of psychotherapy with trauma survivors, to know what it is that needs to be worked on. It is this view of the organism's nature that separates, ontologically, PCT from other forms of therapy such as psychoanalysis and behaviour therapy. PCT is based on this assumption that the organism can be trusted to move in a socially constructive and personally growthful direction. As such PCT is a form of therapy which can help people not only overcome the adverse effects of trauma but also to move towards posttraumatic growth, as illustrated in a later session with Denise:

> Session 16
>
> Cl: We're going away for a few days in the summer, just to a caravan. It's the first time for a while and I feel really good but I'm also worried. Going away brings back lots of difficult memories, everything we used to do always ended terribly. Like I'd be looking forward to something, telling myself things would be good, they may even be a new start or something. Then it would all just be awful and things seemed to get worse than before. Like expecting it to all go wrong.
>
> Th: So a feeling of both looking forward to getting away but also a feeling of dread, like something looming ...
>
> Cl: That's it ... I feel dread right in the pit of my stomach and then surging into my throat, feeling sick. Urggh!
>
> Th: OK, like the feelings are there [points to stomach] and then surging right up here [points to throat].
>
> Cl: Right, and I know they're to do with what's happened. I'm feeling like I want to have some control over these feelings ... I feel I do have some control. Like now we're talking about it and I felt those feelings like right down in the pit and then I felt sick in an instant. But then when you were talking I was just telling myself that that was how I used to feel when I was with him, and I'm not now. Does that make any sense?
>
> Th: Let me check my understanding, so it's like you want to and maybe even do feel like you have a bit more control over feelings that come when you get reminded about the past. Like you feel right now you were able to control a feeling in the pit of your stomach and that sick feeling that followed it.
>
> Cl: Yeah, that's it ... sort of ... I mean coming here and talking has helped put things back together in way I hadn't thought of before. Like I hadn't really thought about me doing the best I could let alone saying that I perhaps did OK to come through all that abuse and still be here now ... like I feel

OK about me when I'm feeling weak with Nick and feeling strong about the past. Or vice versa; I've like got a different take on things now.

Th: So things seem a little different now and you're feeling more accepting of the different ways you feel about yourself.

Cl: Yeah, and I'm feeling differently about what's happened too. Like I can see now that it wasn't my fault, like I understand myself now. I felt ashamed for a long time and that meant I didn't want to talk to anyone or let them know what had happened. But when things started to affect how I am with Nick I started feeling guilty about letting the past affect him. That was when I decided to come get some help and figure things out a little more clearly.

Th: Ah, so these different feelings led you in different directions, like feeling ashamed seemed to lead you away from other people and feeling guilty led you towards getting someone to talk to, is that what you're saying?

Cl: I knew when I was feeling ashamed I didn't speak with anyone because I was frightened. My whole self felt useless and helpless. I thought if I said anything to anyone I would lose the kids, get locked up or something. I felt like I couldn't tell anyone and I used to just feel totally worthless. But when I saw things going bad with Nick it felt a bit different. I felt more able to do something, maybe because he's a child and in some way I knew it was my responsibility; I don't know, not quite figured that out yet.

Th: OK, so the feelings still seem a little confused in how they're helping you find a way forward but it was like the guilty feeling was driving you to do something and you really felt this sense of being responsible to change things with Nick.

Cl: Yeah, I think with him I knew that none of it was his fault and I didn't want my stuff to get loaded onto him, I had to do something and I really feel like things have got much better. I really feel like our relationship is growing and benefiting from me looking back at what happened. I'm not so troubled by it now either ... I get less nightmares now.

In this session we are able to see how the thoughts that act as reminders about the trauma are accompanied by strong emotional and feeling responses. On this occasion it is apparent how Denise is symbolising her experiences. They are accurately symbolised as memories of past events with some apprehension about the trip away. The accurate symbolisation is described as being and feeling more in control and subsequent attributions to the feelings are able to be made that do not trigger further traumatic memories but instead give way to even greater sense of agency. Developing a sense of agency is a core characteristic of posttraumatic growth as people realise that while they cannot change the past, the future is theirs to shape (Joseph, 2011).

Denise is clearly showing signs of posttraumatic growth as she is moving towards integration, with less defensiveness regarding past events and her self-regard continues to extend further and further to all parts of her self-concept unconditionally. She also describes her relationship with her son as benefiting from the integration of traumatic experiences. There is no further description of breakdown and disorganisation as there was previously. Perhaps most interesting is the description by Denise of her understanding of how her feeling responses were guiding her actions and behaviours. She states quite clearly that the experience of guilt was a primary source of motivation for seeking help and of how feeling ashamed had in the past maintained a sense of worthlessness and helplessness and a fear of asking for help. The development of her relationship with her son and of her new outlook on life and self-understanding illustrate how, in working through the meaning of trauma, personal change and growth can arise.

Conclusion

Throughout these excerpts it is possible to see that at no point is the therapist trying to make the client do anything specific. In PCT the therapist's task is to create the environment that is conducive to growth; to experience unconditional positive regard and to communicate this through empathic reflections and statements that are the result of following the client's moment-by-moment experiencing. As we have seen, this approach to therapy places PCT in the position of being a radical ontology for trauma, based as it is on the assumption that the organism can be trusted to move in a socially constructive and personally growthful direction under the right social-environmental conditions. This position remains a radical departure from, and an alternative to, current therapies selected and recommended in treatment guidelines and statutory healthcare provision in the sense that it is the client and not the therapist that determines the direction of the therapy.

The implication of this is that the therapist goes with the client at their pace and in their direction. This may often mean following the client in the way described above with Denise, but we would emphasise that it does not exclude the use of techniques and exercises when they are instigated by the client. Elsewhere we have a presented a model of affective-cognitive processing of trauma that shows the points at which various techniques and exercises may be useful (Joseph, Murphy & Regel, 2012). For example, psycho-education, talking to the client about coping skills, or relaxation exercises can all be helpful. For us the use of such techniques and exercises can support a person-centred approach to trauma therapy, but only if they are used in such a way that respects the self-determination of the client. At some point clients may wish to confront their memories of what happened. Exposure is likely to be helpful. But to introduce such exercises and techniques from the framework of the therapist is not person-centred and in our view not necessary.

> What sets client-centred therapy apart from other therapeutic approaches is the theoretical stance that the client will be motivated by the actualizing tendency to accurately symbolize his or her experience ... the theory holds that the traumatized client will intrinsically be motivated to do this for

him- or herself in his or her own way and at his or her own pace when
the therapist is providing the appropriate social-environmental conditions.
(Joseph, 2004, p. 113)

Finally, the person-centred approach is concerned with facilitating clients to
become more fully functioning. The range of ways in which people become
more fully functioning following trauma are well described by the concept of
posttraumatic growth which we think provides a useful contemporary framework
consistent with the person-centred approach.

References

American Psychiatric Association (APA) (2013) *Diagnostic and Statistical Manual of Mental Disorders* (5th ed). Washington, DC: American Psychiatric Association.

Brabbins, L, Regel, S, Joseph, S & Murphy, D (2013) Inside the filing cabinet of specialized traumatic stress service. Paper presented at British Association for Counselling and Psychotherapy Annual Research Conference, Warwickshire, UK, 11th May.

Grant, B (2010) Getting the point: Empathic understanding in nondirective client-centered therapy. *Person-Centered & Experiential Psychotherapies, 9*(3), 220–35.

Joseph, S (2003) Person-centred approach to understanding posttraumatic stress. *Person-Centred Practice, 11,* 70–5.

Joseph, S (2004) Client-centred therapy, post-traumatic stress disorder and post-traumatic growth. Theoretical perspectives and practical implications. *Psychology and Psychotherapy: Theory, Research, and Practice, 77,* 101–20.

Joseph, S (2005) Understanding posttraumatic stress from the person-centred perspective. In S Joseph & R Worsley (Eds) *Person-Centred Psychopathology* (pp. 190–201). Ross-on-Wye: PCCS Books.

Joseph, S (2011) *What Doesn't Kill Us: The new psychology of posttraumatic growth.* New York: Basic Books.

Joseph, S & Linley, PA (2005) Positive adjustment to threatening events: An organismic valuing theory of growth through adversity. *Review of General Psychology, 9,* 262–80.

Joseph, S & Linley, PA (2006) Growth following adversity: Theoretical perspectives and implications for clinical practice. *Clinical Psychology Review, 26,* 1041–53.

Joseph, S, Murphy, D & Regel, S (2012) An affective-cognitive processing model of posttraumatic growth. *Clinical Psychology and Psychotherapy, 19*(4), 316–25.

Murphy, D, Archard, PJ, Regel, S & Joseph, S (2013) A survey of specialized traumatic stress services in the United Kingdom. *Journal of Psychiatric and Mental Health Nursing, 20,* 433–41.

Rogers, CR (1951) *Client-Centered Therapy: Its current practice, implications and theory.* Boston: Houghton Mifflin.

Rogers, CR (1959) A theory of therapy, personality, and interpersonal relationships as developed in the client-centered framework. In S Koch (Ed) *Psychology: A study of a science, Vol. 3: Formulations of the person and the social context* (pp. 184–256). New York: McGraw-Hill.

Person-centred therapy with adult survivors of childhood sexual abuse

2

Jan Hawkins

Until recently, survivors of childhood sexual abuse would rarely announce themselves at the beginning of a therapeutic relationship. Instead they would begin therapy for such difficulties as depression, anxiety, self-harming, eating disorders, addictions, anti-social behaviour, posttraumatic stress disorder and sexual dysfunction (e.g., Putnam et al., 1986; Scott, 1992; Miller & McCluskey-Fawcett, 1993; Mullen et al., 1993, 1994; Peters & Range, 1995; Romans et al., 1995; Fergusson et al., 1996, 1997; Silverman et al., 1996; Wonderlich et al., 1997).

Over the past 15 years, as the Survivor movement has become more visible, men and women now seek therapy specifically recognising the fact that their experiences of sexual abuse as children are having long-term effects. Part of this shift has been a gradual change in understanding in the general public about with whom responsibility for child sexual abuse rests. When the prevailing socially accepted theory was that of Freud (1896/1958), that is, sexual abuse is either a fantasy the child has, or the child has 'seduced' the adult (usually male) into sexually abusing them, survivors were terrified of admitting what had happened to them as children. Along with Freud's erroneous theories, the prevailing myth was that if you were abused you would go on to abuse. This terrified survivors into silence and also resulted in many avoiding contact with children for fear of harming them.

The focus on female-as-victim and male-as-perpetrator meant that the feminist movement's re-interpretation of sexual abuse simultaneously placed responsibility for abuse on the perpetrator and retained the idea that only girls and women are abused and only boys and men perpetrate abuse (Nelson, 1987; Rush, 1980). Whereas girls and women have been empowered to break their silence about sexual abuse, boys and men continue to under-report. Those services that exist to address the needs of adult survivors continue to focus on the needs of female survivors whilst there are far fewer services for male survivors. Unless and until the vulnerability of both genders and the potential in both genders to sexually abuse little girls and little boys is recognised, there will be limited success in keeping children safe. It is for this reason that, whenever I write about abuse, I use both pronouns to ensure that the focus is on survivors of abuse, whatever their gender.

The work of David Finkelhor (1984, 1986) and colleagues has led to the recognition that, for abuse to happen, someone has to want to do it. Finkelhor's traumagenic model has allowed survivors to begin to place responsibility for their abuse on the person who perpetrated it. Others, for example, Sanford (1991), highlighted the erroneous thinking that has led to the myth that those who were abused will go on to abuse. Data on people prosecuted for abusing children demonstrates that a high percentage of them have suffered abuse themselves as children and the idea developed that a cycle of abuse down the generations was the norm. There are no reliable statistics on those who do not appear in records as abusers. However, it is known that those who recognise the harm they suffered, rather than inflicting harm on their own or other children, in fact choose to enhance the lives of others through such professions as nursing, medicine, social work, therapy and so on (e.g., Miller, 1991; Sanford, 1991). In the UK, the Cross March of 1995 resulted in the delivery of a petition to the Prime Minister demanding a change in the law in the Statute of Limitations. Survivors from all over the country marched in the centre of London, speaking out and finding solidarity in a desire to heal and to bring their abusers to justice. UK law was changed – survivors won an important victory.

Previously, any individual had only three years from the time an injury was inflicted to make a prosecution. After the Cross March campaign, survivors of childhood abuse now have three years to report and prosecute from their 18th birthday or three years from the time they recognise the damage done by the assault. Because of this change and the courage of men and women who have experienced sexual abuse, more survivors are speaking out and seeking therapy to help them recover.

Research consistently demonstrates that exposure to childhood sexual abuse (CSA) appears to increase the risk of psychiatric disorders by approximately two to four times against those of people not exposed to CSA (for a review of studies, see Fergusson & Mullen, 1999). Carmen et al. (1984) found that 50 per cent of psychiatric in-patients reported histories of physical or sexual abuse.

Adult survivors of childhood sexual abuse might appear in psychiatric services for treatment with an eating disorder, an alcohol problem, self-harming, sexual dysfunction, difficulties concentrating, not being able to know who they are, or living with a sense of unreality. These and other symptoms then become the pathology and the individual is trapped in the revolving door of mental health services because these services mostly attend to the symptoms rather than the cause.

Adults who were sexually abused as children have been disempowered. When a child is abused, early supportive intervention will mitigate long-term consequences. When a child feels able to tell a trusted adult that something sexual has happened to them which was confusing, coercive, painful and/or frightening, the child is already showing signs of having a secure relationship with the adult to whom they divulge this information. In those circumstances supportive action can be taken to help the child understand whose responsibility the abuse is and recovery is enabled. However, when a child does not have such a secure relationship, or has been so frightened and/or confused by their abuser and experiences that they are unable to seek help by disclosing, the child is vulnerable to repeated abuse. The child adapts in a variety of ways in order to survive, yet some of these adaptive behaviours cause more harm. The child is vulnerable to re-victimisation in part because they have learned how they must be to survive – how they must behave or what they must do for the abuser. Children in homes where there is persistent threat in the form of violence, sexual abuse, perpetual verbal denigration and assault – in short, where there is chronic trauma – develop coping strategies that help them survive.

These strategies can become so habitual that it is impossible, as adults, to let go of them when the threat has long passed. Some children survive by becoming 'good girls/boys' who never complain, never make demands and attempt to anticipate the adults' every need, having received the idea that their existence depends on being 'good'. Some children survive by lashing out at others, involving themselves in crime; these children are the visible ones, though sadly their self-esteem is further damaged because of the negative attention they draw to themselves. Other children survive by squashing their feelings by, for example, denying themselves food. What is anorexia saying? 'I have no needs.' Or by developing a binge–vomit cycle, that is, swinging between 'I have overwhelming needs', and 'I have no needs'. Alternatively, the survivor overeats in vain attempts at comfort, or anaesthetises her- or himself with alcohol or other drugs. Yet more children develop a creative coping strategy of dissociation – often pathologised, but of all coping strategies the one that is the most invisible. All these coping strategies can be viewed as distress flares (Hawkins, 2003). These and other coping strategies are evidence of distress, but far from bringing in the rescue services, they serve to alienate people further from sources of comfort for their pain. Children whose sexual development has been derailed by the abuse of another person can find it difficult in their adult lives to separate sex from affection or from fear.

It is the possibility of relationship and relational depth (Mearns & Cooper, 2005) that makes person-centred therapy (PCT) particularly potent for people who are recovering from sexual abuse. Sexual abuse does not happen in a vacuum; there is always accompanying emotional abuse in the form of coercion, threats to remain silent and the betrayal of trust. The misuse of power in sexually abusing a child leaves deep and long-lasting wounds which need a reparative, trustworthy relationship to heal (Thorne, 1998, 2002).

For a therapeutic relationship with survivors of sexual abuse to be healing in this way, it is important that the therapist has acquired particular knowledge and understanding of the experiences of those persons who are often diagnosed with 'dissociative identity disorder', 'psychosis', 'posttraumatic stress disorder' and 'complex posttraumatic stress disorder'. This will enable therapists to better understand experiences of dissociation, the differences between psychotic experiences and experiences of flashbacks, and the positive coping involved in self-harming behaviour. In this way they are better prepared to receive survivors of sexual abuse with authentic unconditional acceptance.

In my view, imparting such knowledge and understanding to counselling trainees should be a part of training programs in PC counselling. There are those, however, who disagree with this view, pointing out that PCT means you do not need specialist training as the core conditions are both necessary and sufficient for change to occur (e.g., Rogers, 1957; Bozarth, 1998). The apparent contradiction here may perhaps be overcome by pointing to the deepening of empathic understanding and acceptance gained by being open to, and exploring, a whole variety of experiences; a point that is hardly disputed.

Case study

What follows is an illustration of the darker edges to which therapists may need to accompany clients who are survivors of sexual abuse. The focus is on the experiences rather than the content of this particular case and all possible identifiers have been omitted for anonymity. None of what follows below can be considered in any way prescriptive as each instance of intervention is necessarily idiosyncratic both to the individual therapist's practice and to the particular situation with the client. However, I believe this example illustrates the many boundary issues that often come to the foreground in work with this client group. Issues, which, as this case demonstrates, can go as far as blurring the distinction between the professional and private area of a therapist's life and issues that usually require very supportive supervision for the therapist.

Mary was in her mid-forties when she came to see me. A physiotherapist with responsibility for running a department, she had very recently had a crisis, which had rocked her to the core. Her experience was of suddenly feeling as if she were dissolving into tiny atoms. Sharing this anxiously with a colleague had meant she was fast-tracked into a psychiatrist's office and diagnosed with having a psychotic break and put on medication. It was a month after this that she came to see me as she was not feeling any better and had begun having flashbacks, nightmares and panic attacks. The medication was making her feel worse and she gradually weaned herself off it, but the other symptoms were becoming severe. Despite this, she was working and able to manage work, but when at home she felt she was losing her mind. From the time she arrived until the time she completed her work with me, I was aware that I had never walked so closely alongside a client who so keenly wanted to die. Each time she left, often pausing to sway at the top of the steps, I suppressed the urge to bring her back in. I was holding on to my trust in her at the same time as endlessly revisiting the dilemma of the contract of confidentiality I discuss with every new client, 'if yourself, or another is at risk of serious harm' etc. I have never breached confidentiality, but walking closely with a client who is actively suicidal has never been less than anxiety-provoking in me.

> Does the counselor have the right, professionally or morally, to permit a client seriously to consider ... suicide as a way out, without making a positive effort to prevent this choice? (Rogers, 1951, p. 48)

In our early sessions, Mary described the sensations she was experiencing, in particular the feeling of dissolving. I have had experiences of dissociation from a variety of descriptions from clients and from my own personal background. Exploring what was happening before and after these sensations helped Mary to recognise the triggers, which were always sudden breakthroughs of memories and body sensations. Though we never did know what had triggered the onset of the crisis for Mary, she had always known her history of childhood sexual abuse. She had always remembered, yet never with any feelings attached; her memories were simply the narrative of her life but had never before had any connection for her with her adult life.

She was a high-flier and had a responsible job where she was comfortable in delegating to others and enjoyed the respect of her team and her own line-managers. Her private life had never felt good. She lived alone and had craved, but never had, a relationship with romance, security and children. It seems that she had managed her life thus far by living two separate existences. At work, she was efficient and quick-witted, generally getting on well with her colleagues and patients. At home, she felt dull, sometimes bored and often lonely. She was alive at work but at home she had just slept or kept up with a few friends. During the time of her crisis, everything in her private life seemed false, including her friends, and she withdrew into herself, though she continued to work throughout the 18 months we worked together.

In many of the sessions, Mary seemed dissociated, silent, unresponsive, pale and sometimes scowling as she looked down at the floor. At other times, her thoughts of ending her life were to the fore. At these times, I would stay alongside, listening to her plans and acknowledging the depths of despair she was feeling. Yet I also held that part of her that clearly wanted to live – the Mary who talked about her plans to live in the countryside, to find a life partner and to continue to develop her career.

These two forces were ever present and I asked the life-desiring Mary how she could protect herself from the plans of the desperate Mary. We discussed a commitment that she would telephone me if she were going to end her life with the understanding that I would not be trying to prevent her from doing so, but would be there to hear, bear witness and to ask how the life-desiring Mary felt about it.

There is something about the bleakness and solitude when despair is active and desperate that can feel like there is nothing but darkness and pain to look forward to, that the world would be a better place without you, where the thought of being able to lay down the burden of life is so enticing, it obliterates any other thoughts and feelings. I felt I was working at the edge in every session with Mary and I think I will always remember those sessions. However, two encounters made a particular impression on me, and each was enormously transformative. The first involved a repeated flashback Mary would have in the sessions where she would dissociate into frozen silence.

In previous sessions, she had been able to utter an occasional word. At other times, she had been able to report what had happened after she had emerged from the flashback. We had developed a signal, which let me know what was happening. The particular repeated flashback was of being raped as a young child on a table. Each time I had used every possible means of establishing psychological contact, using contact reflections (Sanders, 2007) that focused on her frozen defensive posture, on the terror on her face, on her breath-holding. At the same time, I was attempting to reassure her that it was not happening now, that she was safe with me and I was there to help her ground back into the real room with me. On the occasions that she was able to respond, I had been able to continue to reassure her as well as inviting her to let me know what she was seeing and feeling. She experienced her abuser as often in the room with us and my acceptance of the normality of this had been helpful to her in her more-grounded moments.

During the course of the sessions, Mary had been able to process many of her traumatic experiences, yet the same flashback of being on the table had the power every time to terrorise her. She reported that, of the flashbacks that she had every night at home, this was the worst. She was terrified of going to bed where she knew she would be raped again (in flashback) by her abuser. Because the flashbacks were related to the age of below 7, we were able to explore in her grounded times what a 7-year-old might need to feel safe in her room at night. We talked about the magical thinking with which children are blessed and talked about creating a force field at the bedroom door so that her abuser could not get in. We talked also about taking the young child out to find a safe protector and as a consequence she came back with a toy rhinoceros and developed a phrase, 'Get him Rhino', to chase away the abuser when other flashbacks and memories arose. Still we returned to the table in sessions and still she was frozen in terror.

In the session which stands out most in my mind, Mary reacted like never before or since. I had attempted to establish contact via contact reflections, but she was too far away. I continued with the assurances of safety. Suddenly I felt that I was in the scene with her (which is not unusual) but that I was somehow complicit; I was watching her being raped and doing nothing about it. I found myself saying firmly 'get him off; he has no right to do that to you, get him off'.

No reaction. I have many cushions in the room and I put one on her lap and again said, 'push him off, fight him off'. Nothing. I placed another and another cushion on top of each other and continued firmly to encourage her to push him away. When all eight cushions were on top of her and there was still no reaction from the terrified frozen woman-child, I thought I had completely lost the plot and may have made things worse for her. I took the top cushion off her and with all the force I could muster, I threw it on the floor and again said 'push him off; he has no right to hurt you'. Suddenly she began screaming and flailing about, cushions flew everywhere, and she continued to flail and scream, landing in a heap on the floor. When she had stopped screaming and begun to weep quietly, I brought to her 'Big Ted' with whom she had bonded in other sessions.

Big Ted is a large bear who sits wisely and quietly in my room. Over the years, he has occasionally become very important to a client. I have never introduced him, but for some clients he just seems to work. Because Mary was quite attached to him, and because of the turmoil she had just been through, I brought him to her and let her know I was covering her with the fleece blanket that is also occasionally useful. Mary could not be touched, which is why these comforters felt important. We were, surprisingly, able to finish our session on time, and we had made contact with the physiotherapist in her who would get her home and keep her safe.

I reflected constantly over the following week on this almost bizarre intervention. Bizarre for me, a person-centred therapist who focuses on the client's frame of reference and allows the client to self-direct! Yet something more powerful had taken over – if I had left her in her own frame of reference, I believe she would have continued to re-live the rape on the table with no way of freeing herself.

When Mary came the following week, she reported that she had not been raped at night (in flashback) since the last session! In reflecting again on this transformative session, I cannot imagine the same thing could have happened if I were to use that same intervention as a routine technique – or earlier in the sessions. It was somehow imperative that it emerged spontaneously in that particular session, even though we had visited that flashback so many times. The release from that particular flashback meant that other memories were processed in less traumatic ways for Mary. She had fought him off and won once, and that changed things. Mary was still suffering and reporting much of the suffering rather than feeling it in the sessions. This dissociative processing is very difficult for survivors as they can so easily find themselves trapped into reliving traumatic scenes or experiencing overwhelming feelings when alone – just like when the original abuse happened. When undergoing therapy, the functioning self is able to take over and simply report on things, which can leave the person very frustrated. Clients like Mary will tell me of the pain, distress and terror they experience at home alone, and fear that, as they are aware that they are reporting rather than feeling in the sessions, I may disbelieve them. For survivors of childhood abuse, these experiences in isolation can feel like a repeat of what happened when they were tiny and conveying the fullness of their feelings with the therapist may seem impossible. Yet there is a yearning to be able to fully express, and not to be alone with the feelings. This leads to frustration and often a sense of never being able to share or to be 'a good client'.

Another encounter with Mary took us to a different edge and was really the pivotal point in the whole therapy. Mary had felt suicidal since the moment she felt herself dissolving and was diagnosed with psychosis. She felt her whole life as a professional woman was slipping away and she suffered terribly with the flashbacks and in particular with the feelings associated with them.

One evening, I was cooking dinner when my phone rang. Picking up the receiver, I recognised the robotic emotionless voice as one of Mary's dissociated selves saying, 'You said I should ring you if I was going to kill myself …'. She had taken herself up on a pylon not far away, and remembered what we had agreed some months before. Thinking on my feet, I ignored the robot and appealed to the professional physiotherapist in her to come and collect a tape I had made for her. The tape was one of my voice (as she could not cope with strangers' voices) talking her through a breathing and anxiety-reducing exercise, which was ready for our next session. I said I would have about 10 minutes if she would just come and collect the tape. Amazingly I had reached a compliant part of her, and she came.

While waiting for her to arrive, I needed to prepare my young son. I would not have seen clients when he was there without either my husband or a babysitter for him. That evening, my husband was due to be home as I had an evening client. But there was no one for my son at that point. So I told him that I had to see someone for 10 minutes (he was used to the sanctity of the therapy room and the no-disturbance rule), and that the client might be upset and not to worry. Being a very mature chap, and being heavily involved in a computer game, he nodded sagely. When Mary arrived, she looked dishevelled and unusually had clearly been crying, and she was now crying very loudly as I took her into the room. The crying reached wailing level and showed no sign of abating. I sat at her feet as she screamed, wailed, sobbed uncontrollably, and I made soothing noises. After a while I became concerned that my young son might be frightened by the level of distress he must be hearing, so I told Mary I had to leave the room for a few minutes but would be back. She was not really in contact with me at that point, but I had to check with my son. He seemed to be taking the noise in his stride! I then asked him to phone my husband and ask that he come straight home as I had a client in distress. My son again sagely nodded and picked up the phone.

Going back to Mary, the distress continued with much screaming, much wailing, tears and snot dripping onto the floor as she hunched over. I knelt by her with the tissue box to which she was oblivious. After about an hour, I began to think I had gone too far, that I might have to call in the mental health crisis team. I would certainly, I feared, have to leave the room again to try to cancel my client who was due in 45 minutes. I went through a variety of feelings during that outpouring of distress; it felt imperative to be alongside her and metaphorically to hold her in all of it. I knew, from other sessions, her greatest fear was that, if she began screaming, she would never stop. I wondered what the neighbours might think was going on … I was concerned about my young son, though I had heard my husband arriving home towards the end of the hour. I prayed for Mary. I thought of R.D. Laing's (1965) authentic state of madness – this must be one dimension of it. Eventually though, Mary's distress quieted and she noticed the tissues and began using them as she continued to cry. She asked for Big Ted and I brought him over. She apologised … It felt like we had been to her Hell and come back from there. I was struck again by how important it was to her that I trusted her to look after herself. I asked some grounding questions: What had she got to eat this evening? What would she watch on television? (A useful distraction for her.) As she swayed on the top step, I again realised how close to the edge we had gone.

Our work continued for some months, but the breakthrough had been and gone. She had been able to scream out some of the terror, the indignation, the humiliation, the pain – and to do that not on her own, but with a companion who could bear witness. Before we completed our work, she had realised some of her dreams and found a lovely little flat in the countryside, and a job in a local physiotherapy practice. On our last session, she brought along 'Rhino' to meet me. As I write this now, some years since we worked together, I can still feel how moved I was by her bringing 'Rhino' along. The significance of the toy was huge. The physiotherapist in her thought that this was a very silly idea when I first suggested that she take her younger self out to choose a comforter but she was very surprised by the power of that experience as it just had to be 'Rhino' and no other.

Without an understanding of dissociative experiencing (Warner, 2000), the nature of flashbacks and their re-traumatising power, I fear I may not have been able to give Mary the companionship she needed to heal. Our relationship was multi-dimensional and I have found Charles O'Leary's (1999, 2012) concept of 'multi-directional partiality' helpful in ensuring that I listen to, and value, each part of the client who has endured childhood sexual abuse. Throughout our work Mary directed the pace and content of sessions, and I endeavoured at all times to use her own language, whichever part of her was present at the time. I was moved, in that relationship, to extend her frame of reference in terms that were beyond her awareness and may always have stayed that way. For example, after a session in which she had been another self, I would ask how she was getting home, what she would do there, what she would eat that evening and so on. For Mary these grounding questions encouraged her to value herself and to take care of herself in ways she had never really considered. The major challenge, however, was to listen closely to her expressions (including the silent ones) and to trust her process rather than becoming tied up with the diagnosis with which she had arrived.

I had moments of doubt when I wondered if I were simply a naïve charlatan who really should have accepted the psychiatric view of Mary. I had moments too where I feared that the responsible thing to do would be to request her psychiatrist's details so that I could liaise with him. Had she requested that of me, as some other clients have, I would have explored that with her and worked alongside her psychiatrist to ensure transparency. But Mary had felt let down and judged by the psychiatrist she had seen and was terrified that she would be sectioned if she shared anything of what she was experiencing with him. So after that first meeting she had had with him, where she had been diagnosed and prescribed medication, she saw him every six weeks for 10 minutes to discuss her medication. She never did tell him that she was weaning herself off the medication until she was feeling stronger towards the end of the therapy. Her fear that I too would think that she was psychotic, or worse, would silence her at times. Her courage to risk telling me those fears and what she was really experiencing left me then, as now, in a state of awe.

What Mary valued most, she told me at the end of our work, was my trust in her and my recognition of the strength the professional Mary had, at the same time as recognising the terror of the younger Mary who needed to have a witness to what she had suffered. Having always known what had happened, but never before her crisis having felt it, when she did begin to experience the fear, it led to the feeling that she was losing her mind; yet that is when she was becoming more herself (Rogers, 1961/1967). When we completed our work together and said goodbye, she shyly gave me a tiny ornament, which continues to sit in my therapy room. I have heard from her from time to time. Though she has had occasional blips where she feared revisiting her crisis, she has come through them and life is good. Our work took me truly to the edge and confirmed my passion for offering the relational depth and what I can only describe as soul accompaniment of the person-centred approach to healing and recovering from childhood sexual abuse.

Conclusion

Since the Cross March of 1995 in London and awareness-raising campaigns, more survivors are speaking out. It is now not uncommon to have a potential client ask about the potential therapist's experience and training in the area of sexual abuse. My advice to those seeking a therapist to help them heal from the legacy of childhood sexual abuse is that they ask the therapist 'Whose responsibility is child abuse?' If the therapist wavers, she or he is not ready to accompany the client through what can be terrifying terrain as the client heals the wounds from possibly many years ago.

Survivors need trustworthy supporters who have examined their own attitudes, beliefs and experiences, and continue to deepen their understanding of the legacy left by the trauma of childhood sexual abuse. Further, therapists need to ensure that they have support around them and, in particular, a knowledgeable and experienced supervisor who is able to encourage and support the therapist during what can sometimes be long-term work. It is the relationship that heals, and as I consider those I am currently accompanying through the process of healing, I am again humbled by the courage it takes to find the words to place the terror outside of themselves and into the room for me to witness. For some, the silence has been tightly maintained for many, many years, sometimes held down by heavy drinking or drug use.

> And then the day came when the risk to remain tight in a bud was more painful than the risk it took to blossom. (Anaïs Nin, cited in Sanford, 1991, p. 35)

Person-centred therapy offers the depth of relating and trust in the client's own self-directed process to provide the reparative experience of real empowerment. As survivors develop their emotional muscles in exposing their deepest pain, it behoves us, their therapists, to continually work out our own emotional muscles to provide the accompaniment they deserve in their healing.

> Congruence and compassion open the way to using what Kopp (1974, p. 3) considers to be the therapist's primary instrument in healing: 'the personal vulnerability of his own trembling self'. (Wosket, 1999, p. 214)

It is a continually striving to remain genuine, transparent and accepting of the darkest of actions taken in distress that allows therapists to bear witness and therefore be alongside the client as he or she heals the wounds left by those who have treated them as an object for their own gratification. The person-centred approach has particular dimensions that facilitate healing: a real relationship is available and the client is empowered to direct her or his own process. Everything about abuse means that the child has been completely disempowered, and feels helpless and defenceless. Any therapeutic approach which, in any way, replicates these feelings by putting the therapist in the powerful position of directing what 'should' be explored, or by interpreting the client's motivation, rather than encouraging the client to explore and learn more about their process and connect more with their inner self, is at risk of replicating the harm caused. It is the relationship that heals.

References

Bozarth, J (1998) *Person-Centered Therapy: A revolutionary paradigm*. Ross-on-Wye: PCCS Books.

Carmen, EH, Ricker, RP & Mills, T (1984) Victims of violence and psychiatric illness. *American Journal of Psychiatry, 141,* 378–83.

Fergusson, DM, Horwood, LJ & Lynskey, MT (1996) Childhood sexual abuse and psychiatric disorders in young adulthood. Part II: Psychiatric outcomes of sexual abuse. *Journal of the American Academy of Child and Adolescent Psychiatry, 35,* 1365–74.

Fergusson, DM, Horwood, LJ & Lynskey, MT (1997) Childhood sexual abuse, adolescent sexual behaviours and sexual revictimisation. *Child Abuse and Neglect, 21,* 789–803.

Fergusson, DM & Mullen, PE (1999) *Childhood Sexual Abuse: An evidence-based perspective.* Thousand Oaks, CA: Sage Publications.

Finkelhor, D (1984) *Child Sexual Abuse: New theory and research.* New York: Free Press.

Finkelhor, D (1986) *A Sourcebook on Child Sexual Abuse.* Beverly Hills, CA: Sage.

Freud, S (1958) The aetiology of hysteria. In J Strachey (Ed and Trans) *The Standard Edition of the Complete Works of Sigmund Freud* (Vol 3, pp. 191–221). London: Hogarth Press. (Original work published 1896)

Hawkins, J (2003) 'Softly, I can do it softly.' In S Keys (Ed) *Idiosyncratic Person-Centred Therapy: From the personal to the universal* (pp. 37–50). Ross-on-Wye: PCCS Books.

Laing, RD (1965) *The Divided Self.* London: Pelican Books.

Mearns, D & Cooper, M (2005) *Working at Relational Depth in Counselling and Psychotherapy.* London: Sage.

Miller, A (1991) *Banished Knowledge.* London: Virago.

Miller, DAF & McCluskey-Fawcett, K (1993) The relationship between childhood sexual abuse and subsequent onset of bulimia nervosa. *Child Abuse and Neglect, 17,* 305–14.

Mullen, PE, Martin, JL, Anderson, JC, Romans, SE & Herbison, GP (1993) Childhood sexual abuse and mental health in adult life. *British Journal of Psychiatry, 163,* 721–32.

Mullen, PE, Martin, JL, Anderson, JC, Romans, SE & Herbison, GP (1994) The effects of child sexual abuse on social, interpersonal and sexual function in adult life. *British Journal of Psychiatry, 165,* 35–47.

Nelson, S, (1987) *Incest: Fact and myth.* Edinburgh: Stramullion Co-operative Ltd.

O'Leary, CJ (1999) *Counselling Couples and Families: A person-centred approach.* London: Sage.

O'Leary, CJ (2012) *The Practice of Person-Centred Couple and Family Therapy.* Basingstoke: Palgrave Macmillan.

Peters, DK & Range, LM (1995) Childhood sexual abuse and current suicidality in college women and men. *Child Abuse and Neglect, 19,* 335–41.

Putnam, FW, Guroff, JJ, Silberman, EK, Barvan, L & Post, RM (1986) The clinical phenomenology of multiple personality disorder: Review of 100 recent cases. *Journal of Clinical Psychiatry, 47,* 285–93.

Rogers, CR (1951) *Client-Centered Therapy: Its current practice, implications and theory.* Boston: Houghton Mifflin.

Rogers, CR (1957) The necessary and sufficient conditions of therapeutic personality change. *Journal of Consulting Psychology, 21*(2), 95–103.

Rogers, CR (1967) *On Becoming a Person.* London: Constable. (Original work published 1961.)

Romans, SE, Martin, JL, Anderson, JC, O'Shea, ML & Mullen, PF (1995) Factors that mediate between child sexual abuse and adult psychological outcome. *Psychological Medicine, 25,* 127–42.

Rush, F (1980) *The Best Kept Secret: Sexual abuse of children.* New York: McGraw-Hill.

Sanders, P (2007) *The Contact Work Primer: An introduction to Pre-Therapy and the work of Garry Prouty.* Ross-on-Wye: PCCS Books.

Sanford, L (1991) *Strong at the Broken Places: Overcoming the trauma of childhood abuse.* London: Virago.

Scott, KD (1992) Childhood sexual abuse: Impact on a community's mental health status. *Child Abuse and Neglect, 16,* 285–95.

Silverman, AB, Reinherz, HZ & Giaconia, RM (1996) The long-term sequelae of child and adolescent abuse: A longitudinal study. *Child Abuse and Neglect, 20,* 709–23.

Thorne B (1998) *Person-Centred Therapy and Christian Spirituality: The secular and the holy.* London: Whurr.

Thorne, B (2002) *Mystical Power of the Person-Centred Approach: Hope beyond despair.* London: Whurr.

Warner, MS (2000) Person-centred therapy at the difficult edge: A developmentally based model of fragile and dissociated process. In D Mearns & B Thorne (Eds) *Person-Centred Therapy Today* (pp. 144–71). London: Sage.

Wonderlich, SA, Brewerton, TD, Jocic, Z, Dansky, BS & Abbott, DW (1997) Relationship of childhood sexual abuse and eating disorders. *Journal of the American Academy of Child and Adolescent Psychiatry, 36,* 1107–15.

Wosket, V (1999) *The Therapeutic Use of Self: Counselling practice, research and supervision.* London & New York: Routledge.

Person-centred therapy with people with learning disabilities: Happy people wear hats

3

Jan Hawkins

I offer you peace. I offer you love. I offer you friendship. I see your beauty. I hear your need. I feel your feelings. My wisdom flows from the Highest Source. I salute that source in you. Let us work together for unity and love.
(Mahatma Gandhi)

Gandhi's message could not be more relevant to the experiences I have had when working with people who are differently abled, cognitively challenged, learning disabled. In this chapter, I shall discuss briefly the terms of reference regarding people with learning disabilities and lay out my belief, born of long experience, that the person-centred approach can be a particularly good 'fit' for responding therapeutically to individuals with this label. I shall then offer some illustrations through the therapeutic relationships I have had with people with learning disabilities. All identifying details have been removed to ensure anonymity, and some details have been changed for the same reason. My purpose in sharing such case histories is to encourage other therapists to develop their confidence in offering therapy to people who may not speak, or whose communication is very different to the 'neurotypical'. 'Neurotypical' is a term used by autistic people to describe non-autistic people. Though the term has only been in use for about 10 years, it does collectively describe the majority of people whose cognitive, social and functional abilities allow them to develop along a common trajectory and to live independently as adults who also share a theory of mind, about which more below. Using the term 'neurotypical' allows us to move on from using the term 'normal'.

Terms of reference

Definitions of learning disability have changed many times over the years (see, e.g., Sinason, 1992). The terms have not generally been chosen and owned by people with disabilities themselves. Often the descriptive terms that are used are principally to do with how resources are allocated. Definitions based upon intellectual ability, legislative definitions and social competence have variously been used to try to define a group of the population who do not, usually due to congenital issues or birth difficulties, share the same cognitive abilities as the neurotypical population.

The World Health Organization has defined learning disabilities as: 'A state of arrested or incomplete development of mind' (WHO, 1992, p. 7).

For the purposes of this chapter, I shall discuss my work with clients who have already been given a diagnosis of learning disability or severe learning disabilities and with autistic spectrum disorders (ASD). All of these clients have lived either in residential homes, supported living or with parents or carers. None of them have been sufficiently able to care for themselves and live independently, and so they rely on the people around them for their daily needs. The clients with whom I work and who have these 'diff-abilities' (Edmonds, 2012) may or may not be able to use verbal or even sign language.

The challenge for me therefore is to develop consistently my ability to attune to each unique client's communication, whether verbal or non-verbal. Clients who do not conform to the received tradition of the 'talking' therapies challenge their therapists to consider where boundaries may need to be flexible; you may need to reconsider the time boundaries to allow for the differing needs and affinities of individuals from this client group (Hawkins, 2002); you may need to extend your skills by learning Makaton[1] or BSL (British Sign Language) to facilitate communication; your patience may be challenged and even your idea of what constitutes therapy or what beneficial use of therapy looks like. More so than with neurotypical clients, you will need to let go of any notion of end product – process is all; you may need to be able to converse about soap operas, children's books or sales catalogues; you may need to consider the best interests of the client in sharing any learning from therapy sessions in the form of recommendations for care staff. These and other challenges face therapists who want to offer an inclusive therapeutic service. And throughout all of this, we are challenged always to reflect on our deeper attitudes to, for example, 'who has a right to life'.

For person-centred therapists who regard the relationship as central to the therapeutic endeavour, we are challenged to walk our talk even more than with our neurotypical clients who, at least to some degree, we can assume have a shared theory of mind (Baron-Cohen, 1995).

Theory of mind (ToM) means the ability to recognise and understand thoughts, beliefs, desires and intentions of other people in order to make sense of their behaviour and predict what they are going to do next. Baron-Cohen, (1995) describes ToM as a form of 'mind reading' in the neurotypical world and the difficulties that people with ASD have in understanding others as 'mind blindness'.

---

1. Makaton is a language programme designed to provide a means of communication to individuals who cannot communicate efficiently by speaking (e.g., Grove, N & Walker, M (1990) The Makaton Vocabulary: Using manual signs and graphic symbols to develop interpersonal communication. *Augmentative and Alternative Communication*, 6(1), 15–28).

When we are working with people from different cultural contexts than our own, we need to develop an understanding of the norms and expectations, accepted behaviours, traditions and also learn a different language. For those who are not cognitively impaired, and are within our cultural contexts, we can rely on certain shared understandings and norms of behaviour. We can also rely on our verbal abilities to make communication at least a possibility. For clients who do not have that shared theory of mind due to living with ASD (Baron-Cohen, 1995), or whose learning-disabled culture and living circumstances as well as cognitive functioning are very different from the general population, we are challenged fully to enter a different emotional and cognitive landscape, and that can lead to feeling de-skilled and sometimes helpless. These are not comfortable feelings with which to sit and may interfere with the ability to suspend our own theory of mind in order to really understand the world of our client, who sees and feels things very differently. My experience with many of the people with learning disabilities I have met, and especially those within the autistic spectrum, is of a refreshing honesty and lack of façade. An example of this happened in a choir I was leading, made up of volunteers, parents, staff and people with learning disabilities and autism. At our first, and most resplendent, concert, the Mayor and various dignitaries were present along with the press. As the leader of the choir, I was asked to have a photograph taken with said dignitaries, and a microphone was there for me to say a few words about our wonderful choir. At this very moment, as the audience waited, no doubt in great anticipation, one of our choir members stepped forward and announced loudly: 'But Jan, you're not photogenic, are you!' I could only respond: 'I suppose I'm not.' Fortunately I find this kind of straight talking refreshing, though having the microphone there was taking things a little too far!

Clients who have ASD and/or the range of learning disabilities have even fewer opportunities than those who are neurotypical to develop ways of experiencing and communicating their emotions. In fact, to be able to connect with their own experiencing, they may need the stimulation of their carers (Pörtner, 2007) and also their therapists. At the very least, they need someone who is really paying attention to what they are trying to communicate.

Sadly, people with learning disabilities, severe learning disabilities and/or ASD are often only able to access a limited range of psychological supports, in the UK predominantly in the form of behaviour modification programmes or cognitive behaviour therapy. Sometimes the focus of this work can be spending time observing them and talking to staff or parents, with the therapist less often being able to have the time to develop a relationship with the client themselves and thereby learn what the person's distress or sometimes very challenging behaviour may be expressing. Emerson and Einfeld (1995) suggested that challenging behaviour:

refers to behaviour of such an intensity, frequency or duration that the physical safety of the person or others is likely to be placed in serious jeopardy, or behaviour which is likely to seriously limit use of, or result in the person denied access to, ordinary community facilities. (p. 7)

The nature of care and support for adults and children with learning disabilities in the UK is such that therapeutic support is sometimes only considered when the individual's behaviours present serious difficulties to those who are supporting, caring for, or teaching them. Terms like 'challenging behaviour' or 'challenging needs' refer to challenges posed to the people around the client, but the behaviours expressed are communicating something. We must ask ourselves whom the behaviour is actually challenging.

Carl Rogers (1951), Alfred Adler (1938/1998) and others have asserted that all behaviour is purposeful and best understood as a person's way of coping with the problem rather than the problem itself: 'Behavior is the goal-directed attempt of the organism to satisfy its needs as experienced, in the field as perceived' (Rogers, 1951, p. 491).

If those of us hoping to help people with learning disabilities do not endeavour to understand what their behaviours, however challenging, are communicating, we have no real hope of helping them make changes. We need: '… to see with the eyes of another, to hear with the ears of another, to feel with the heart of another' (Adler, cited in Ansbacher & Ansbacher, 1964, p. 135) and understand: '… that human beings flourish best when they can experience acceptance and understanding rather than adverse judgement and a lack of informed responsiveness from others' (Mearns & Thorne, 2000, p. 15).

Case illustrations

I have had a number of sessions involving walking with a client, allowing him or her to lead whilst I had no idea where we were going. For the clients I have accompanied on these walks, I was acutely aware of their sense of purpose in striding forth and I knew, in each case, that these clients never went out of their day centre or home unaccompanied and rarely had the opportunity to lead. Their walks, in general, were to and from the minibus or to and from specified activities. For a client who could not even decide to get up and go out for a walk without a carer present, having me alongside seemed to be an unusual experience.

Jake

Jake is gaze-averse, finding any face-to-face interaction extremely difficult, if not impossible. So walking alongside allows some of the strain of interaction to drop away. I am constantly attempting to tune in to where he is as we walk. After a while of simply walking alongside in silence, I start offering 'contact reflections'

(Prouty, Van Werde & Pörtner, 2002; Sanders, 2007). For those for whom mumbling and disconnection is their predominant mode of interaction, these walking sessions offer the opportunity for occasional pauses, and I can make temporary psychological contact. A relationship of this order allows the client to connect (Adler, 1938/1998) and that increases the desire for connection. In such 'sessions', I am able to offer real acceptance, and my empathy can be demonstrated on a number of levels, for example, keeping pace with Jake and allowing him physically to lead demonstrates rather than talks about the possibility for directing his own process. Having said that, if Jake did not eventually turn towards the day centre or home, I would need to let him know that we were expected back and that I would need to leave him back where we started. Yet, oddly enough, that has never happened with Jake or the others with whom I have had walking sessions. In these sessions, I cannot claim that I have *done* anything with the person, nor addressed the concerns that have led to the referral. Yet the experience of being alongside someone who is not attempting to guide them onto a minibus or into an activity may still be very unusual for these people.

I have found that our connections, however brief, deepen over time and without actually focusing on it, the particular behaviour of concern sometimes diminishes.

Following are three case illustrations where the edge has been different in each case. The clients were not able to refer themselves for therapy, but each was referred by a member of the support team caring for them. This means that these three clients had already benefited from the consideration and care of staff, who could tell the client was distressed, or causing distress to others, and were willing to do what was necessary to get a referral.

Gary

Gary is a man in his fifties with severe learning disabilities. Though he has a functional language and a reasonable vocabulary, he often lapses into repetitive noises, teeth clamping and repetitive phrases. He has a history of challenging behaviours in that he can become very agitated and hit out at people. He has been referred by the team supporting him as they consider finding him a new place to live. They have decided to see if therapy might help him to settle in a home as he had already moved house 11 times in the past 13 years. The reason for these moves, in the main, is Gary's repeated refrains: 'I want to move', and 'I don't like it where I live'. I learnt quickly during our sessions that when repeating these phrases, Gary becomes increasingly anxious and agitated. It is difficult to re-establish psychological contact with him during these times and he will often get up from his chair and loom over me anxiously repeating the phrases. Gary challenges me in other ways too; I have to ensure that I have protected the chair on which he always sits as he is frequently doubly incontinent and leaves a considerable smell in the room. In order to remain accepting and not find myself reacting to this smell, I always have a candle lit during his sessions – he likes that very much whilst not knowing why it is there! After his sessions, I have to open the windows and wash the cover I have used for the chair. Gary enjoys a cup of coffee, which I always offer him when he arrives. He has been on the minibus from the day centre for quite a time, and making the drink for him allows him some quiet time in the room, and he clearly seems to enjoy that; I often find him relaxed with his eyes closed when I come in again with his drink.

From the first session, Gary was repeating his 'I want to move' refrain. During the early sessions, I aimed to track him very closely in his utterances, using contact reflections (Prouty, Van Werde & Pörtner, 2002; Sanders, 2007), word-for-word reflections, reflections about his body posture and guesses at feelings. The loop in which he gets caught would resolve when he would eventually say: 'I phone social worker tomorrow, he sort it out'. I could understand why the team were finding the repetitions difficult to cope with, and also why they had decided to simply ignore Gary when he began these agitated loops. However, they had also clearly been trying to act on Gary's obvious anxiety, and had been moving him from flat to flat, house to house, and residential home to residential home over the past 13 years. I knew from the referral that the pattern was always the same: Gary would agree he wanted to move into each place, would say it was alright for the first few weeks, then begin again to insist that he wanted to move. In an effort to empower him, they had continually moved him on. Another move was imminent when he came to me. During the course of the therapy, I gradually began to understand Gary's predicament. The last time he had liked where he lived was when he lived with his mum and dad. Gary's experience of family life sounded to have been a very positive one, where he felt comfortable and safe. Since his mother died, he had not found another attachment figure and understandably missed her terribly. Gary knew Mum had been ill but did not go to her funeral and so did not know where she was, though he did say she had died.

In my experience, being able to say that someone has died does not always mean the person has a concept of what having died means. During this series of sessions, we talked more about his life with his mother especially. It seems she worked in an office and Gary sometimes went to work with her. He used to visit his sister and her family with Mum. He and Mum also visited her friends. They would have meals together, watch TV together and she would give him a cuddle when he was upset. With Mum's death, Gary had lost contact with all the friends he used to visit with her, as well as his sister and her family. Gary seemed to think he had brothers too who he would visit with his mum, but he could not remember their names. Putting myself where Gary had been, the happy and secure family life he had enjoyed until he was in his forties had suddenly been lost. Not only had his mother died but his contacts with his siblings and his mother's friends had all stopped, and Gary was living in one place after another, always saying he was unhappy there. We talked about his parents and the loss of his family home, and also the loss of the family holiday home in Eastbourne, which the family frequented, as well as the loss of his father's Mini and the opportunities he had to drive it. Apparently his father would take the Mini onto a private piece of land and let Gary steer. I was struck by the sudden devastating losses Gary had endured. During one session, he said, 'I like it here, it's a home', speaking of the room in which we sat during his sessions. It was at this point that I fully realised why Gary insisted he keep moving. He was looking for home, looking for the comfort and security he had felt at home where Mum and Dad would have meals with him and watch TV. In most of his moves, he either lived alone or with one or other persons with learning difficulties. Support workers would come in for a certain number of hours each day and Gary would go to the day centre during weekdays. He told me that at weekends, he would stay in bed. Gary continues to repeat: 'I want to move', and 'I don't like it where I live', because he is searching for the comfort and familiarity he felt when living with his parents.

As we came to the end of the agreed 10 sessions, I discussed with Gary what he wanted to share with his support worker and social worker. He was able to say that he wanted a home and that he missed his mum and dad. I find it pains my heart to be fully with someone like Gary, whose concept of death is lacking in any real understanding. When his dad died, his mother was able to tell him, and he still had her. Later when his mum became ill and went to hospital, he has no memory of visiting her there. He was clearly informed when each of them died, but did not attend the funerals. Suddenly his home, his companionship, his whole life disappeared and he began the endless search for peace and comfort.

The team supporting Gary asked me to advise on his next placement, based on what I had learned from him. Gary and I talked with his support worker about finding him a home with a family, where he could be part of a family. He would have carpets on the floor and a sofa. He would like someone who would watch TV with him sometimes and talk with him. I suggested that, rather than finding yet another supported living placement, they find an adult fostering placement. It was at this point that Gary and I said goodbye.

About a year later, Gary returned for a few more sessions. He had begun his repeated 'I want to move,' and 'I don't like where I live' refrain fairly soon after moving into a house with a family who had agreed to foster him. In this series of sessions, we talked about what he liked about where he was living – there were, indeed, carpets! He liked having the clean clothes and his washing done for him. He liked not having to make his own packed lunch or other meals. He liked that the mother of the family did these things for him. He liked his room and he liked the people who would talk to him sometimes. He felt lonely: the family were not speaking English all the time, so he felt confused. He always had his meals alone rather than with the family at their table. Having the space and attention to express what he was feeling, Gary gradually calmed in the sessions and his repeated, agitated phrases reduced to only about three or four times each session. Whenever he repeated them, I would now respond with variations of 'you are really missing your old home', or 'it's not the same as with Mum and Dad' – some acknowledgement of what he was really feeling. Here was the edge. Gary is unlikely to ever feel comfortable and easy again. The love and comfort he enjoyed with his family have gone and whatever is put in place for him, it cannot replicate that.

My hope was that sharing the last session with him and his support worker, where I modelled responding to Gary's repeated phrases, would help the support worker to recognise what was lying at the heart of Gary's continued requests to move. I shared my feeling that some training for the people who were supporting Gary would be most helpful in recognising earlier his rising anxiety, and in developing some empathic responses that allowed him to feel understood. I also recommended some support for those members of the team who felt they should be finding him a new place to live every time he became agitated and repeated these phrases endlessly. It is hard to think life can never be made comfortable for Gary. However, he does respond and calm when he is met fully in that terrible sadness.

Kim

Kim was referred to me by the residential home in which she was living. In her mid-thirties, she had always previously been relatively calm and compliant. She was now causing difficulties in the home she shared by having explosive outbursts where she would smash furniture, and whenever possible, the television. Kim had very little verbal language and severe learning disabilities. It took several sessions for us to make any meaningful contact. Like many of my clients, one highlight for her was having a cup of tea when she arrived. Her journey from the residential home to me was over an hour, and a cup of tea was clearly always very welcome. She settled with her support worker leaving her, even in the first session, and showed no sign of wanting to leave early. Her support worker would say that she was going to the café for a cup of tea. I would follow up with, 'and we can phone on the mobile if you want her to come back early'. I don't believe that Kim understood these words in any clear way, but I do feel she had a sense that the phone would bring back her support worker. Her utterances were extremely few and far between, and I aimed to catch each and show her I had understood. Fairly quickly she showed some interest in the colours and paper I had, so I brought these to her. She was always very still. It was hard to imagine Kim suddenly exploding and smashing things. In an effort to establish and maintain contact with her, I began drawing what she said, and this did encourage her to say more.[2]

---

2. I have found that having drawing materials at hand can facilitate communication for those people with whom I work where verbal communication is limited. Having something to draw on or to simply touch and hold can help some people with learning disabilities to express themselves where words do not come easily. At times too, I find that picking up the pencils myself and drawing what the person is saying creates a connection between us.

Much was disjointed. A name, or words like car, fire engine, hat. My drawing skills would probably be assessed as approximately those of a 4-year-old. Despite this, I have managed a semblance of whatever she was saying. Whenever I drew, she showed more interest in connecting with me. She liked to take the drawings with her, so I found a folder and we would clip in each session's drawings, and she would take them away and bring them back. As another way of connecting, I asked her support workers for photographs of staff, residents, her family and the rooms where she lived. Kim loved to go through these pictures in sessions and her utterances increased.

In one session, I noticed that she was particularly upbeat and used the word and sign for happy. She did use a few signs, and this seemed to be a new one for her. So I drew a circle with a smile and signed and said: 'happy'. On the same paper I drew a sad face and signed and said: 'sad'. She seemed very interested in this and I was reminded of other clients with whom I have worked who seemed never to have been given a way of saying how they felt. Kim would refer to these drawings in subsequent sessions – and we developed them with the addition of 'angry'. Though the support workers who would bring Kim to her sessions would sometimes report that another 'incident' had occurred, Kim remained calm and still in our sessions. I had managed to compile a list of her utterances related to the happy, sad and angry drawings. I made three cards about 3-inch square. Each had one of the faces, and on the back of each I wrote the things Kim had said which related to those feelings. Having laminated them, I punched a hole through each and fixed them on to a key ring. I have found these key rings to have a variety of uses in my work with people with learning disabilities, in particular as methods of task building. In this situation, I was hoping that Kim might use them to show her support staff what she was feeling – they could then run through the possibilities on the back of the card to see if one fitted what Kim wanted them to know. Kim did take to this and seemed delighted with her key ring. This prompted me to make another, with all the people in her life, from a set of photos I had requested. She absolutely loved this set and would often want to run through them in sessions. These photos were especially helpful when she wanted to tell me something about someone, and I was struggling to understand.

So the sessions were useful, but had done nothing to help the explosive incidents at home. Then one day, as we sat together on the sofa while I drew Kim's disconnected thoughts, there was a noise outside. People were walking past in the street shouting at each other. We could not see them as the room is above the street, but we could hear them. Kim suddenly moved in a way I had never seen. She instantly jumped and began shaking. Before this could go any further, I announced firmly: 'Those people are shouting, but they will not come in here. You are safe here, they won't come in.' She calmed a little. I was able to encourage her to sit. That was when I drew the 'frightened' picture to add to her key ring. It felt to me as though Kim was having a panic attack. I talked in a very slow, soothing voice, and focused on contact reflections, 'your hands are shaking', and so on. I also showed her how to breathe really slowly, all the while reminding her that no shouting would come into the room.

Following this session, I asked the support staff to review the incident reports for what had been happening before Kim had exploded and smashed things. None of the incident reports recorded what was happening before, so I asked that they make a particular effort to record what was happening before, during and after any further incidents. We continued our sessions and it was not long before a pattern emerged. Kim's explosive behaviour was happening when the BBC TV soap opera *EastEnders* was on the television. It became apparent to me that she was frightened when the characters became angry or shouted – quite a frequent occurrence in that particular programme. I suggested that Kim have one-to-one support when watching *EastEnders* from then on. I offered guidelines for recognising rising anxiety and how to reassure Kim that no shouting would happen in the room, that she was safe and that the staff would look after her. Kim's uncharacteristic outbursts had shocked the support staff where she lived and what seemed to be their view was that she was going through an angry and destructive phase. In fact, she was frightened and felt threatened by the sound of angry voices and was relatively easily calmed. Empathy in the moment and reassurance was all that was needed. Using a behaviour modification response, i.e., removing her from the room after one of her incidents, would only serve to reinforce her distress. Kim needed in-the-moment anxiety management support. As the staff became more skilled in this, and more confident in their abilities to spot rising anxiety and help Kim to calm, things improved for her.

In our last session Kim and I looked through her collection of drawings and I noticed a theme I had not spotted before. She was always interested in hats – my attempts to draw them were always rather odd, but she was always satisfied. I noticed that all the smiling stick figures, whose names she had insisted I write, though she could not read, were wearing hats. None of the angry or sad faces had hats on. I remarked to her that, 'happy people wear hats', and she nodded enthusiastically. What that means or meant, I have never really discovered as she was not able to tell me, but her slow-to-get-it therapist had got there in the end! What was important to Kim from our sessions was not whether or not she was having explosive incidents at home, but whether I actually knew what she was trying to say, whether it meant anything to me or not. To this day I find that humbling.

Richard

I have written elsewhere about Richard (Hawkins, 2003). In his early fifties, he had severe learning disabilities and I had seen him over the course of some years at the day centre where I offered a day a week. Like so many others, Richard had been 'dispersed' (King's Fund, 1999; Thompson & Mathias, 1999) into the community from a long-stay hospital. His story had come out in tiny fragments over those years and was one of extreme physical abuse at the hands of some of the nurses whose job it was to care for him. Living in the community in a house with others with whom he had not chosen to live and with unfamiliar support staff caused Richard, like many others I worked with, considerable confusion. He had lived his life in an institution. Not a safe or happy life, but one with which he was familiar. I have often wondered if the politicians who decreed the great 'dispersal' into the 'community' of people in long-stay hospitals had ever spent any time with the people they were helping. Whilst to most of us, a choice between living in a hospital ward and living in a house in the community would be easily made, for the clients I have worked with and who have been moved into the community, choice was not any part of the deal. Richard was simply given his packed bag, put on a minibus and taken to his new house. In his long-stay hospital, he had been used to wandering around the grounds and going to the day centre and back by himself. In his house in the community, a minibus picked him and others up to take them to a day centre a 20-minute ride away.

During the time we worked together, Richard had been able to articulate, between confabulations, episodes of violence he had endured in the hospital, like being taken into the 'domestic cupboard' and beaten with the vacuum-cleaner hose for example. He sometimes recited an address, which I learned from the support staff at the day centre was the address of his family home. Richard, again like so many other clients with learning disabilities, had not been to his mother's or father's funeral. He seemed vaguely to know they had died, yet often pondered aloud where they could be. Part of our work involved me helping him to understand the concepts of death, not coming back, and missing them. The reason Richard springs to mind now, as I write, is that he and I went to an edge together. We went to the confines of his fear and despair. He was able to share with me, in very disjointed ways, what was happening at the home in which he lived. Inappropriate behaviours from staff towards another resident were frightening Richard. He was becoming more and more distressed – 'high' was the word used by support staff in reporting to me Richard's increasingly challenging behaviours. I had explained in various ways, in the hope he really would understand, that I had to speak to his social worker about what was happening. Of course, he verbally consented – but what does that really mean for someone like Richard? The misuse of power he had endured throughout his life had made him try very hard to figure out what the 'right' answer was, and to comply. This kind of dilemma faces us when working with vulnerable adults. I did make the referral to his social worker.

What happened next will stay with me always. Richard was medicated, heavily medicated. When I saw him for the last time, he hardly knew me. And then he disappeared from the day centre and it took some weeks for me to learn what had happened to him. Richard had been taken into a locked psychiatric ward where he stayed. The report on the home in which he had lived received superficial attention and nothing changed in that home according to the day centre staff. Richard was a casualty. His challenging behaviours had to be dealt with for his own and other residents' protection. He was a gentle soul, but hugely distressed. So the focus was on dealing with the symptoms and not the cause. For Richard, seeing what was happening in the home, the punishments the staff was meting out on other residents, was triggering distress and fear from the memory of what had happened in the hospital. And I seemed completely impotent to do anything other than my referral. As his therapist, it was all I could do to raise the concerns. But Richard was a vulnerable adult whose testimony would not be taken seriously as his communication had needed the fullest of my attention to comprehend. I learned some months later that Richard had died in the psychiatric locked ward. His suffering was never relieved, but we did meet on the edge and I comfort myself that in those moments, he did feel connected.

Conclusions

Working therapeutically with people who have severe learning disabilities requires patience. It also requires us to let go of any of our own needs to be powerful. In many ways, it is even more humbling than working with others whose suffering brings them into therapy. We must look for the tiniest sign of movement. With the core attitudinal qualities of the person-centred approach, growth does occur. But it is unlikely that a person with severe learning disabilities will transform into someone without them. People with severe learning disabilities rely on others to ensure that they are fed, clothed, housed and have a life of meaning. They cannot do it alone. This can mean that the efforts made in the therapeutic relationship are possibly the only times in their lives that clients like Jake, Kim, Richard and Gary receive full attention and efforts to understand them. Support staff are often underpaid and trained to focus on practical care needs rather than on understanding the communication, verbal and non-verbal, of the people they support. We are challenged then to consider how we can best serve our clients with severe learning disabilities. I continue to hold the dilemma and discomfort whenever I share something with a support worker who has asked about my work with a client with severe learning disabilities. I have to trust myself that whatever I do share is in the best interests of the client. Though I always discuss what I might think would be helpful to share, I know that my clients with severe learning disabilities have had no power in their lives over what is communicated about them. My desire to have an impact for them has brought me to the conclusion that the best help I can be is to work with the client for enough sessions to develop an understanding of their inner world and their feelings. I then want to work with their support staff in training. Not to share any content from the sessions, but to share my understandings of what is happening for the client and how they may best be supported.

In training support staff, I am keen to flush out those who come with a punishment agenda. Sadly some support workers regard the people they are supporting as either 'naughty' children or wilfully 'misbehaving' and needing to be 'taught a lesson'. Sometimes staff workers freely admit, for example, that they make a resident wait till last for his cup of tea, because he did something 'naughty' earlier in the day.

Staff workers with a punishment agenda in a team undermine the work of the rest of the team. For people with severe learning disabilities even more than for neurotypical people, consistency is all-important if change is really to take place.

Used in this way, the person-centred approach can make real differences in people's lives. What is on offer for people with severe learning disabilities who are in distress is psychological support, usually in the form of behaviour management plans. But these can never truly address this condition. Unless we understand what the behaviour is communicating, we cannot understand the person. If we want to enable and empower the person, rather than manage him or her, we need to open our hearts and minds to understand.

> If I accept the other person as something fixed, already diagnosed and classified, already shaped by his [or her] past, then I am doing my part to confirm this limited hypothesis. If I accept him [or her] as a process of becoming, then I am doing what I can to confirm or make real his [or her] potentialities. (Rogers, 1961/2004, p. 55)

References

Adler, A (1998) *Social Interest.* Oxford: Oneworld Publications. (Original work published 1938)

Ansbacher, HL & Ansbacher, RR (Eds) (1964) *The Individual Psychology of Alfred Adler: A systematic presentation in selections from his writings.* New York: Harper and Row.

Baron-Cohen, S (1995) *Mind Blindness: An essay on autism and theory of mind.* Cambridge, MA: MIT Press.

Edmonds, C (2012) 'Diff-ability' not 'Disability': Right-brained thinkers in a left-brained education system. *Support for Learning, 27*(3), 129–135. Article first published online 18 September 2012. doi: 10.1111/j.1467-9604.2012.01524.x

Emerson, E & Einfeld, SL (1995) *Challenging Behaviour.* Cambridge: Cambridge University Press.

Gandhi, M Quotation retrieved 20 November 2012 from www.quotes.net/quote/13209

Hawkins, J (2002) *Voices of the Voiceless: Person-centred approaches and people with learning difficulties.* Ross-on-Wye: PCCS Books.

Hawkins, J (2003) 'Softly, I can do it softly'. In S Keys (Ed) *Idiosyncratic Person-Centred Therapy: From the personal to the universal* (pp. 37–50). Ross-on-Wye: PCCS Books.

King's Fund (1999) *Learning Disabilities: From care to citizenship.* Retrieved 23 November 2012 from www.kingsfund.org.uk

Mearns, D & Thorne, B (2000) *Person-Centred Therapy Today*. London: Sage.

Pörtner, M (2007) *Trust and Understanding: The person-centred approach to everyday care for people with special needs* (2nd ed). Ross-on-Wye: PCCS Books.

Prouty, G, Van Werde, D & Pörtner, M (2002) *Pre-Therapy: Reaching contact-impaired clients*. Ross-on-Wye: PCCS Books.

Rogers, CR (1951) *Client-Centered Therapy: Its current practice, implications and theory*. London: Constable.

Rogers, CR (2004) *On Becoming a Person*. London: Constable. (Original work published 1961)

Sanders, P (Ed) (2007) *The Contact Work Primer: An introduction to Pre-Therapy and the work of Garry Prouty*. Ross-on-Wye: PCCS Books.

Sinason, V (1992) *Mental Handicap and the Human Condition: New approaches from the Tavistock*. London: Free Association Books.

Thompson, T & Mathias, P (Eds) (1999) *Lyttle's Mental Health and Disorder* (2nd ed). London: Harcourt.

WHO (World Health Organization) (1992) *The ICD-10 Classification of Mental and Behavioural Disorders: Clinical descriptions and diagnostic guidelines*. Geneva: WHO.

'Tenuous contact': New theory about adolescent process | 4

Peter Pearce and Ros Sewell

This chapter describes meeting the challenge of connecting adult counsellor to adolescent in the counselling relationship within a school environment. It charts the development of a proposed new concept, 'tenuous contact', arrived at by the authors after more than 10 years' counselling within secondary schools. The authors believe the term 'tenuous contact' most accurately reflects the sometimes fleeting and 'fragile' style of contact that can be part of the counselling relationship with young people. 'Tenuous' captures the notion that the counselling relationship is sometimes difficult to obtain and feels hard to maintain, and it also makes sense to many parents and teachers in terms of their relationships with this age group. The authors are from a person-centred tradition and in this case, requiring to be 'young-person-centred', they decided to take a positive approach to the tenuousness and to explore how to make the most of it for the benefit of their young clients.

The location is an Inner London secondary school; the event is a therapeutic group session with Year 9 students,[1] which takes place on a regular basis. One of the students has struggled to engage for several weeks. This extract illustrates the frequent efforts in this setting to connect with a young person and meet them where they can begin. It is the opening of the session.

> Student: Nothing really ... normal.
>
> Counsellor: It seems really difficult for you to stay with this part of the session each week, the best bit and the worst bit of your week ... is that right?
>
> Student: [silence then angrily] My week's been shit alright?
>
> Counsellor: [gently] Your week's been shit.
>
> Student: Yeah ...
>
> Counsellor: [hesitantly] Any part of your shit week that's been any more shit than the rest?
>
> Student: [long silence] Yeah last night, my Dad come in drunk and hit my Mum.

---

1. In UK secondary schools, Year 9 students are between 13 and 14 years old.

This is our story – and the students' story – about managing and working with 'tenuous contact', which not only offers a way to frame the experience between adult and adolescent but, very importantly, creates an opportunity for the adolescent to reframe their relationship with their own experiencing. We hope to extend the terms and articulation of what takes place when connecting at various levels in this environment and with these young people, as well as inviting a re-evaluation of what kind of contact may be 'necessary and sufficient' (Rogers, 1957; Stern, 2004). Persistence and consistency over time seem to be important constituents which we describe later. We have found through regular contact in our teaching and supervision roles with other therapists that those who work with young people are aware of this fragility in relationships with young people and have been implicitly working with it. They have welcomed attempts to articulate it so that their knowledge and experiences can be more easily shared within the profession, resulting in the development of best practice in this area.

The worlds of a young person and an adult counsellor are often so far apart that real engagement and connection may seem impossible. In the following example, the counsellor is challenged not only by the possibility of not being able to understand the young person's language but by the value references to a different culture that are being expressed.

> Student: [spoken very quickly – almost without a pause for breath] I'm not 'av'n nuffin' to do wiv 'er no more – she fuck'n speak'n to me like tha' – I don't cotch wiv 'er no more – I saw 'er out she's shit right – she fuck'n blanked me – this is me right don't blank me – this is 'er right I weren't – boy she's a liar – I know if someone fuck'n blanks me – know what I mean? – I'm pissed man – and then in school today right – she says she's bringing 'eads down – I'll tell ya – she don't get me shook – if she's bringing 'eads down – I'm bringing 'eads down – I'm bringing bare 'eads down an' we got borers right – d'you get me?

Young-person-centred

Connection with a young person may have to be striven for and the level of the contact may vary from session to session and fluctuate during the session itself.

Striving for contact with young people can at times feel like more than offering unconditional positive regard and trying to stay in their frame of reference. It can feel like *sensing* the threads, thoughts and feelings of their *unspoken* world and holding that sense very gently until they express their experience in sometimes unexpected ways. They might not be able to make sense of their experience at first, but they may be able to put it in a place where it causes them less hurt.

Tenuous contact might, therefore, be thought of as akin to Van Werde's description of 'grey-zone functioning' (Prouty et al., 2002) developed in adult mental health settings. This might be thought of as rapidly changing functioning; sometimes being in good, mutual contact with the person, and, at other times, having little sense of what is going on in them. With young people this experience can be of both being anchored in the shared reality and sometimes also the 'pre-expressive'[2] and sometimes where the two realities are blended together. In Van Werde's terms then, tenuous contact might be situated in the upper half of this grey-zone functioning very close to 'normal' expressive functioning,[3] but partially remaining in a private world. For some this might predominantly be a 'not choosing' to connect with an adult, and for others it may be less of a choice where this 'locked-in' feature has become a way of being.

In either case, as a counsellor with young people you often have to endure the frustration of not yet receiving full contact. Contact has to be 'earned' and may have to be tested – the relationship has to be safe enough for a young person to permit themselves to be in contact with another.

We have noticed that establishing contact can be like a new beginning for each session and the contact gained in previous sessions cannot be taken for granted. Contact for a young person from session to session can feel new, difficult and tenuous. It may not be possible to re-ignite a previous link, which can often be taken for granted at the beginning of a session with an adult. There is no 'relational capital' – at least none that is available in the moment – on which to build.

Young people can frequently be much more in the moment and in order to establish contact a therapist needs to be attentive and sensitive to the mood and expression of the young person at the first encounter. This can be unspoken and a 'tuning-in process' may happen in the transition time, from waiting room to therapy room or in schools, for example, en route from classroom to counselling room.

How did this concept of tenuous contact develop?

This concept emerged during a substantial collaborative doctoral research project that has focused on exploring the impact of 'coming out' of both the real and metaphoric counselling room (Pearce & Sewell, 2008) and being more present in the culture of an inner city secondary school as we searched for the type of school counselling service which might have most impact for students and staff. 'Out of the counselling room' initiatives have included:

- developing a peer-support project
- therapeutic group work

2. In such situations of contact loss it is not always possible to know whether the person has the capacity but is unable to make contact or whether they are consciously withdrawing from contact. This first situation, when someone is capable but unable, is described by Prouty as 'pre-expressive'.
3. Expressive functioning is the psychological state of being when all contact functions are engaged and working fully.

- whole class and year group initiatives to develop emotional literacy
- a programme of counselling skills for teaching staff
- a weekly 'Ask a counsellor' slot on the school radio.

The counselling service was offered in one of London's largest inner city secondary schools with a majority refugee/asylum seeker family intake, more than 100 languages spoken and far greater than usual numbers of students with special educational needs and eligibility for free school meals. In the catchment area, 83 per cent of children under 15 belonged to families that were dependent on unemployment benefits, the highest proportion in any ward in London (London Child Poverty Commission, 2006). The impact of all these challenges meant that many young people arrived with poor literacy and were often displaced and distressed.

In this setting, we found the struggle to connect, for us, for staff, and for students, was stark. We quickly realised that we were not going to get far if we stayed in our counselling 'cultural enclave' expecting others to come to us, to understand and trust what counselling was, and what its benefits could be. We were challenged to translate and adapt our practice and position if we were to succeed in offering something meaningful in this setting. We would have to find a way to carry out research that would help us to provide a counselling service appropriate for the cultural setting. To achieve this we would need to be in regular and open contact with the school structure and staff. To meet some of the challenges that this school setting posed, we kept detailed notes, trying to make sense of our experiencing, which led into beginning more formal, systematic research.

From the notes taken at the time, and from thoughts and issues brought to supervision, the beginnings of 'tenuous contact' can be traced back to the very start of us working together as counsellors within this school. Our early conversations and supervision sessions were dominated by questioning whether what we were actually doing in the counselling sessions with young people was of any value.

We noticed that these supervision sessions highlighted how very different working with young people was from working with adults. We were keen to try to understand what was happening, how we were managing the counselling work in this setting, what was different, trying to identify what exactly we were offering in this context and with what intended impact.

We both kept individual journals and brought aspects of them to supervision for discussion; we recorded some of our reflexive conversations and on other occasions we kept notes. These excerpts have been taken from our work with individuals and groups. The names of the young people have been removed and some narrative details changed to protect confidentiality.

Journal excerpts

M: *So different each session, last session unable to connect and quiet and this week, so easy to connect with. We've noticed that it doesn't always seem to be connected to what has happened to him in the week – still trying to understand this one.*

W: *Really struggled with W this morning, didn't seem to want to be here. Not too sure what is happening at home. Finding sessions with W difficult generally – it seems difficult to make contact with W but not always. Last session really engaged talking about his dad and today so distant.*

T: *Hard to connect again – seems to be in his own world.*

J: *Still not sure what is going on here – J quiet, responds well to any input from us but not really engaging with other students; noticed some connectedness with H when she offered empathy.*

H: (another student member of a weekly therapeutic group we facilitated in the school) *'I saw you coming in with your dad, I didn't know why but I felt sad for you, I knew you were in trouble.' J looked up and smiled, 'It was bare shit man, it's fucking shit.' There's something so clear here about empathy having the ability to touch another and the impact of feeling understood helping them to say more. This was quite a moment in the group. Both of us were able to share our own feeling of being moved by H's empathic reflection and its impact. This encouraged both J and H to share deeply about their own current problems – other participants were also visibly moved within the group. This had a big impact on A who stayed calm enough to bring himself into the room and share his own story about when he had been in trouble for hitting his four-year-old brother. We really recognise the need to record some of this amazing stuff.*

In our analysis of these experiences a repeating theme of 'struggling for contact' emerged and we went to the existing literature to try to find supportive theoretical maps. This sifting of the literature has included exploring the continuing plasticity of the adolescent brain, research into child development and the evolving construction of the therapeutic relationship.[4]

---

4. We have been grateful for dialogue and support from Dion Van Werde, Mick Cooper and Charles O'Leary. Their ideas have helped to shape and develop our own.

Research and literature on adolescence/teen years

Adolescence involves physical, cognitive and social transitions:

- physically, with the onset of puberty, the termination of physical growth and major changes in brain structure and organisation

- cognitively, with improvements in the ability to think abstractly and multi-dimensionally

- socially, as a period of preparation for adult roles.

Piaget (1977) identified how abstract thinking develops through adolescence, enabling reasoning in a wider perspective and prompting a decline in egocentric thought. This theory has support from behavioural and functional magnetic resonance imaging (fMRI) studies showing how the coordination and control of thoughts and behaviour develop through the teen years with the emergence of 'executive functions' (Choudhury et al., 2006).

Neurobiologically, teenage years are a period of rapid growth and development in brain structure and function (Dahl, 2004). The biggest changes during this time take place in the parts of the cortex that process cognitive and emotional information. Some of the most developmentally significant changes are in the prefrontal cortex, which is involved in decision making and cognitive control, as well as other higher cognitive functions (Casey, Jones & Hare, 2008).

Neural connections between this prefrontal cortex and other regions of the brain are strengthened and the efficiency of information processing is improved during adolescence by myelination and synaptic pruning, leading to better impulse control and evaluation of risk (Segalowitz & Davies, 2004). However, relationships between brain and behaviour are complex and adolescent experiencing and behaviour cannot be adequately explained by the continuing development of the prefrontal cortex alone. Casey et al. (2008) argue that the risky choices and actions observed during adolescence represent a non-linear change in behaviour, distinct from childhood and adulthood. A number of studies (Reyna, 2006; Gardener, 2005; Steinberg, 2004, 2005) have shown that adolescents know that they are engaging in risky behaviour and are able to reason and understand the risks, but in the moment this knowledge doesn't stop them. For Casey et al. (2008), this is explained by recent findings suggesting that different aspects of brain structure follow different developmental trajectories. This is particularly the case for the subcortical limbic regions relative to cortical control regions. Galvan et al. (2006) found that adolescents, in comparison with both children and adults, showed a heightened response to anticipation of reward. Casey et al. (2008) suggest that this heightened responsiveness to reward along with the immaturity of areas of impulse control may bias adolescents to seek immediate rather than long-term gains, perhaps helping to explain the increase in risky decision making and emotional reactivity. They put forward a more complex model of adolescent neurobiological development suggesting the need for consideration of 'developmental changes across both context (emotionally charged or not) and time (in the moment or in the future)' (Casey et al., 2008, p. 126). Though it would be fanciful to try to assert some link to our experience of tenuous contact, it is interesting that these areas seem to parallel considerations that have emerged from our own research and experience of adolescent process. It would appear that even when we consider neurobiological development alone, at adolescence we need to think about relationships and environment! It will be instructive to track experiences of tenuous contact against this rapidly developing field of adolescent neurobiology.

Constructions of the therapeutic relationship

Recent years have seen increasing research support for the idea that the quality of the therapeutic relationship is central to the effectiveness of therapy, coming behind only 'client variables' and 'extra-therapeutic events' as a reliable predictor of therapeutic outcome.

The concept of the therapeutic relationship has evolved and developed from Rogers' research-derived assertion of the necessary and sufficient conditions (Rogers, 1957) through the exploration of the importance of the 'working alliance' (Greenson, 1967; Bordin, 1979; Gelso & Carter, 1985), 'presence' (Bugental, 1976; Rogers & Stevens, 1986), the shift to 'mutual intersubjectivity' (Jordan, 1991), descriptions of phenomenological 'moments of meeting' (Stern, 2004) and emphasis on 'relational depth' (Mearns & Cooper, 2005).

Mearns and Cooper (2005, p. xii) describe relational depth as,

> A state of profound contact and engagement between two people, in which each person is fully real to the other, and able to understand and value the other's experiences at a high level ... A reciprocal and enduring sense of contact and inter-connection between two people.

However, there seemed to be a lack of fit between developing person-centred theory and our experience with young people. We found such constructs as relational depth to be less relevant in our work with distressed children and young people – occurring less frequently than anticipated – whilst contact of a more fleeting nature that continually seemed to need to be re-made appeared more commonly. The term 'tenuous contact' emerged to most appropriately describe these therapeutic encounters which did not easily fit in with the accepted theoretical literature originating in work with adults. Some tentative aspects of this construct from our research are described below.

Relational depth as a construct emerges from adult relating. This is not a construct with which many parents of adolescents might identify. Adult–

adolescent relating seems less about relational depth and more about persistence and consistency over time, in short episodes based on the physical and emotional availability of the young person rather than that of the adults. Relationship for a puberty-fraught adolescent seems more often to be about an adult being there somewhere, consistently and non-judgementally.

> Student: It's so fucking boring in here I'd rather be in double Maths! I mean what is this group?
>
> Counsellor: Yeah I've got that, it's so fucking boring that you would rather be in Maths ... and that would be OK.
>
> Student: What would?
>
> Counsellor: Maths, it would be OK if you wanted to go to Maths.
>
> Student: Well I dunno, a bit of me wants to go and a bit of me wants to stay here ... find out if I like it.
>
> Counsellor: You're not sure Donna, you want to go and you want to stay and find out if you like this group ... you know ... both parts are very welcome here Donna.

So tenuous contact might be thought of as relational consistency defined by group; adolescent physical and emotional availability which require non-judgementalism of the therapist; sensitive listening and speaking; reliable persistence; being consistent; being there; no expectations or demands, but a modelling of space boundaries. What's important is the 'contact' rather than the 'content' in each encounter.

Hypothesised causal factors for tenuous contact

Power issues

Within a school environment adults are authority figures whom students see as having expectations of conformity, as judgemental and as having power over many aspects of their lives, including their futures. The students would be right in this perception in many cases.

Third-party referral

It may not be the young person who has the motivation to explore the issues causing concern. To them the concern may be part of the conformity expected, or being judged and told in some way that they are broken and need to be fixed. It cannot be assumed that a young person understands what counselling is for, what is being offered, what the impact will be and how they have to behave to get across this hurdle, as well as all the other hurdles in school life. In a sense these young people may be at the edge of therapy, what the solution-focused brief therapists describe as relating as a 'visitor' to therapy rather than a 'customer' (De Shazer,

1988), or what motivational interviewing constructs as 'pre-contemplation' in the cycle of change (Prochaska & DiClemente, 1984).

Institutional system issues

We have found that individual efforts in this setting can only be fruitful if surrounded and supported by a 'total approach'. This is similar to Van Werde's description (regarding Pre-Therapy work in in-patient mental health settings) of the necessity of translating a set of dynamics into a 'contact milieu' (Prouty et al., 2002). The institutional 'rules', conditionality of the environment, and the hierarchical and conformity aspects of the culture often preclude a sensitive accounting for individual difference and needs, as evidenced in such declarations as, '*He can't come today because he has to do an assessment*', or '*She can't attend counselling today because she's been internally excluded*', or '*Perhaps you can talk to her today in your session about that incident with the pencil!*' Seeing and responding to *this* individual uniquely is the intention of therapy, making them 'exceptional', whereas in school the good practice culture might be concerned with equity, fairness and not making exceptions for one person which might appear unjustifiable to others. This culture clash is also a clash of philosophy of ethics with a utilitarian or consequentialist perspective predominating in many educational settings, where ethics are understood to be concerned with bringing about the 'best' consequences, i.e., the 'best' consequences for the majority of students. In practice this might be interpreted as 'the greater good', justifying the response to any one individual's need (perhaps applying to staff as well as students in some settings): '*Her behaviour (distress) is affecting the learning of the whole class*', as justifying a student's removal from learning and peer opportunities.

In counselling, on the other hand, certainly humanistic counselling, the approach is predicated on a more deontological, or dutiful, view of ethics in which certain types of actions are intrinsically good or bad. For example, telling the truth, respecting autonomy and keeping promises. In practice, a dogmatic embodiment of this perspective has led to criticisms of selfish individuality, holding the individual in mind without properly accounting for their impact on the larger context. This clash of ethics underpinning the differing cultures of counselling and education needs considerable goodwill and openness to adaptation on both sides if these two cultures are to co-exist to mutual benefit within schools counselling.

A clear example of the individual being missed in a rigidly held utilitarian institutional culture happened when a student was distressed about being given detention and was worried about her dad finding out. There had been previous allegations of sexual abuse in the family of which the school was aware. Peter was concerned enough to speak to the newly arrived Deputy Head, who was unaware of any of this history. She told Peter that all students were being given detention for poor behaviour in class. Peter explained the exceptional circumstances, she thanked him for his concern and said that it would be better if she was allowed to do her job and he did his. Peter was under the impression that he was doing his job in alerting her to the special circumstances of this case.

So the school counsellor will likely have to spend time positioning their work in the structure of the institution if they are to address the potential culture clash between counselling and education that can also make the context for school-based work 'tenuous'. A school counsellor may need to find a language to enable them to connect at all levels if their work is to be effective. Not only might both counselling and adult concepts and language need to be adapted to reach young people but a similar bridging/translation process may be needed for the work with other stakeholders such as teachers. Counsellors might find themselves caught up in the 'rhetoric gap' between what is espoused and what takes place within a school structure, as the above example illustrates. The school was keen to establish a counselling service and yet was not able to adapt to the information it provided.

These issues of motivation, understanding, power and context might easily lead to the majority of potential clients being experienced as 'didn't want counselling' or 'inappropriate for counselling'. To model good practice in this setting we believe that a sensitive understanding, both of these context issues and of tenuous contact, is required, alongside a willingness to work at a Pre-Therapy level to build relationship. In this setting, the building of relationship 'is the therapy' and often continues to be required afresh every session.

Possible implications for practice

It seems sometimes as if all previous knowledge of connection and disconnection is 'lost' making it easier for the counsellor to take a position of power. The counsellor needs to be mindful of what has gone before and what the student might not be saying, as the student may start each session as if the relationship and previous sessions had never happened. The counsellor must be aware of this possibility and therefore 'hold' certain aspects of the therapy content and process between sessions.

It may lie with the counsellor to initiate discussion if difficult issues are to be acknowledged, as the young person will rarely bring them back. The counsellor needs to be aware of what has gone before and may need to take sensitive and context-informed risks so that the possibility of a deepening relationship increases.

Moments of difficult contact that have occurred in previous sessions can seem to dissolve as can moments of good connection. It can also be easier to connect after a difficult session. Following a session where one of us had been congruent in the group and some painful insights were gained by a student through some strong challenging on our part, she met us in the corridor the following day and rushed over to speak; it was easy to begin again. We were still in touch with our feelings from the session the day before when we had felt directive and controlling. She brought none of this and at that moment we had a choice, to act as if nothing had happened or to acknowledge that there had been difficulties. We were transparent and said that we were feeling uncomfortable. She responded by saying that it had been a difficult session for her in the group and we all shared how we had experienced it. We felt that we had met her fully at that time and she had been able to be honest with us. It was this exchange that started us thinking about the importance of being transparent and that it was the counsellor's responsibility to bring up any unfinished business or uncomfortable moments. In this example the student was feeling uncomfortable about the previous session but would not have brought it up unless we did. This was an important discovery for us – that an understanding of tenuous contact is important to ensure counsellors do not let moments like this one go unaddressed, believing that there isn't a problem because the student hasn't brought it. We have learnt that, when no sensitivity is shown, power inequalities can be reinforced and may collude with a young person's perception of how unfair adult-to-young person's relating can be.

We have found tenuous contact to be a useful term which has impacted on how we have constructed our therapeutic work with this group to optimise the chances of success. It offers a conceptual framework to support person-centred practice with children and young people. Such practice is a good fit because it strives to stay respectfully within the young person's frame of reference, no matter how present they appear to be, and this can help to narrow the gap of understanding. To borrow from Gadamer (1960/1989), counselling is not a procedure for understanding, but rather for clarifying the conditions in which understanding can take place.

Striving to be phenomenological, that is, to see relationship as a phenomenon and without agenda, can be important since without such a non-judgemental approach something said within the session can sometimes result in lost contact. We have found that the 'presence' sought within a person-centred approach can be unique in the young person's world – a world where some adults may have been either absent or have related on their own terms and have therefore not been able to step into and honour the young person's world as the young person sees it.

Tenuous contact may provide some help with understanding the nature of a therapeutic relationship with a young person, helping describe and explain some of the challenges of working with this client group. Consistency is often the key, so counsellors working with young people need to offer low-level, invitational contact and consistency over time – remaining there, somewhere, on the young person's terms, non-judgementally and often in the background.

This concept values young people and makes them central to the process. It requires specific skills from competent practitioners and locates the establishment of the relationship with a young person on their terms at the heart of the work. Young people are used to adults making relationships 'about them' rather than relationships for use on their terms.

Impact of the concept

We have presented this concept at workshops and at a number of conferences and have been interested and encouraged by the feedback to date – therapists working with young people state that tenuous contact feels like an accurate description of their experience of the difficulties in connecting with a young person in a therapeutic relationship. Some therapists have reported that understanding the relationship in these terms has helped them to feel more positive about their work and stopped them from believing they are 'not good enough' counsellors.

Workshop participants who are parents of teenagers as well as therapists have responded to the concept from a different perspective. They report that this concept makes sense to them and helps them to understand developmentally what is going on for their teenagers and why they sometimes feel they are connected and can speak to their youngsters and sometimes feel that they are not able to approach them.

This chapter is a response to requests from workshop participants to share some initial thoughts and ideas. Further publications exploring tenuous contact in greater depth are planned.

We hope this contribution to the field of person-centred counselling – an approach highly relevant, and appropriate, to work with young people – can help open the door for sharing and development by offering new language to discuss theory and practice development in a rapidly changing world. Therapists are translators and facilitate communication across barriers within a person, between a person and others, and a person and the world. Our hope is that 'tenuous contact' might help others, as it has helped us, both as counsellors working with young people and parents of teenagers, to hang in there with young people when we are unsure of what is going on, to stay with it when we feel de-skilled and useless, and to continue to reach out when we are not sure if anything is being received.

References

Bordin, ES (1979) The generalizability of the psychoanalytic concept of the working alliance. *Psychotherapy: Theory, Research & Practice, 16*, 252–60.

Bugental, JFT (1976) *The Search for Existential Identity*. London: Jossey-Bass.

Casey, BJ, Jones, RM & Hare, TA (2008) The adolescent brain. *Annals of the New York Academy of Sciences, 1124,* 111–26.

Choudhury, S, Blakemore, S & Charman, T (2006) Social cognitive development during adolescence. *Soc Cogn Affect Neurosci, 1,* 165–74.

Dahl, RE (2004) Adolescent brain development: A period of vulnerabilities and opportunities. *Annals of the New York Academy of Sciences, 1021,* 1–22.

De Shazer, S (1988) *Clues: Investigating solutions in brief therapy.* New York: WW Norton.

Gadamer, HG (1989) *Truth and Method* (2nd rev ed) (J Weisheimer & D Marshall, Trans). New York: Continuum. (Original work published 1960)

Galvan, A, Parra, CE, Penn, J, Voss, H, Glover, G & Casey, BJ (2006) Earlier development of the accumbens relative to orbitofrontal cortex might underlie risk-taking behavior in adolescents. *Journal of Neuroscience, 26,* 6885–92.

Gardener, MS (2005) Peer influence on risk taking, risk preference, and risky decision making in adolescence and adulthood: An experimental study. *Developmental Psychology, 41,* 625–35.

Gelso, CJ & Carter, JA (1985) The relationship in counseling and psychotherapy: Components, consequences, and theoretical antecedents. *The Counseling Psychologist, 13,* 155–243.

Greenson, RR (1967) *The Technique and Practice of Psychoanalysis Vol 1.* London: Hogarth Press.

Jordan, JV (1991) Empathy, mutuality and therapeutic change: Clinical implications of a relational model. In JV Jordan, AG Kaplan, JB Miller, IP Stiver & JL Surrey (Eds) *Women's Growth in Connection: Writings from the Stone Centre* (pp. 283–9). New York: Guilford Press.

London Child Poverty Commission (2006) *Monitoring Child Poverty in London.* September.

Mearns, D & Cooper, M (2005) *Working at Relational Depth in Counselling and Psychotherapy.* London: Sage Publications.

Pearce, P & Sewell, R (2008) Applications of the person-centred approach 'coming out' of the counselling room: Holding a psychotherapeutic posture within an educational setting. *Person-Centred Quarterly* (February).

Piaget, J (1977) *The Development of Thought: Equilibration of cognitive structures* (A Rosin, Trans). Oxford: Viking.

Prochaska, J & DiClemente, C (1984) *The Transtheoretical Approach: Crossing traditional boundaries of therapy.* Homewood IL: Dow Jones-Irwin.

Prouty, G, Van Werde, D & Pörtner, M (2002) *Pre-Therapy: Reaching contact-impaired clients.* Ross-on-Wye: PCCS Books.

Reyna, V (2006) Risk and rationality in adolescent decision making: Implications for theory, practice and public policy. *Psychological Science in the Public Interest, 7,* 1–44.

Rogers, CR (1957) The necessary and sufficient conditions of therapeutic personality change. *Journal of Consulting Psychology, 21(2),* 95–103.

Rogers, CR & Stevens, B (1986) *Person to Person* (Reprinted ed). London: Souvenir Press.

Segalowitz, SJ & Davies, PL (2004) Charting the maturation of the frontal lobe: An electrophysiological strategy. *Brain Cogn, 55,* 116–33.

Steinberg, L (2004) Risk taking in adolescence: What changes, and why? *Annals of the New York Academy of Science, 1021,* 51–8.

Steinberg, L (2005) Cognitive and affective development in adolescence. *Trends Cogn Sci, 9,* 69–74.

Stern, DN (2004) *The Present Moment in Psychotherapy and Everyday Life.* New York: WW Norton.

Pre-Therapy at its edges: From palliative care to exercising newly recovered contact functioning

5

Dion Van Werde

Introduction

In 2000, the city of Gent, Belgium, organised an art project called 'Over the Edges'. Artists installed site-specific, mostly open-air art installations, placed at the corners of streets and squares in the city. The idea of the 'edges' was that a city defines itself by its edges. Pivotal places of reference that originate at the crossing or touching of different entities. Places that have significance and function as beacons to the wanderer, to the one that is looking for something to hold on to, to stay oriented in the flood of encountered data.

When writing about Pre-Therapy and contact work, the same idea crosses my mind. Pre-Therapy is a way of offering the client or the person encountered handles to get rooted again amidst the flood of experiences he or she maybe is locked into, or even drowning in. This being said, it is implied that to meet the client, one has to look at the 'edge' where the client's world meets ours, a demarcation area where subtlety is needed in order to be allowed to visit the area or even to be allowed to merely refer to it. Sometimes it is unaccessed territory, even for the person themselves, sometimes vacant – long since abandoned. It is the line where change is possible, where the two worlds clash and perhaps bridges can be built.

Garry Prouty (1936–2009) made the comprehensive term 'contact' the subject matter of his professional life. His experiences with people admitted to vast wards in state mental hospitals with low levels of (if any) psychological care offered, highlighted the problem of how to apply Carl Rogers' insight about the vital importance of the quality of relationship offered, in order to achieve some therapeutic progress (Rogers, 1957). Relationship as such was unattainable with many people who had been locked into themselves for 30 years or more in an institution, with a kind of arrested emotional functioning. Eugene Gendlin (1968) would call it 'frozen functioning': people no longer able to touch a concrete, bodily felt, process of inner functioning. Rather, they were doomed to being locked into repetitive functioning. For example, always being paranoid, no matter what was happening, who they were with, no matter what the season, weather, and time of the day and so on; people unaware of their inner life, not able to find answers in themselves about which choices to make and the nature of their feelings. It is exactly at these edges that Garry Prouty's work is situated (Prouty, Van Werde & Pörtner, 2002). His work can be called pre-relationship and pre-experiencing activity. This implies that the therapist or caregiver enables the person worked with to again reach a point of relationship (cf., Rogers) and experiencing (cf., Gendlin).

Prouty uses Merleau-Ponty's insight (1962) that man is to be defined as a conscious being and consciousness is always intentional. It reaches out to the world, the other and the self: these are the fields of awareness. I am always conscious of something. In a 'pre-expressive' state, these awarenesses, these connections, are troubled, deformed, disenfranchised and the person is left in a kind of existential autism, a state of not-being-in-connection. They are on their own, shielded by a protective bunker of psychological isolation, locked into their own reality.

Garry Prouty no longer saw strange, odd and even bizarre behaviour as totally deprived of meaning and function. On the contrary, similar to a premature baby, these behaviours carry, by definition, a kind of 'not yet mature' quality. A promise of, but still not accessible, meaning and purpose. They have the potentiality to become 'expressive' and meaningful for both the witness and the person who manifests it. They carry content in a 'not-yet' manner. If we pick up the comparison with Rogers and Gendlin, we could say that this pre-expressive behaviour expresses relationship and experiencing on a 'pre-level'. They promise, and have the potency to make a transition to an expressive level – that is, if the circumstances, the nourishment and the right person at the right moment are there. The premature baby will grow and 'mature' if everything offered is matched with the actual level of functioning; milk at a certain age, mashed cooked vegetables later – so to speak. In the same way, if a caregiver finds a way to make a therapeutic offer that matches the level of functioning well, and thus serves and 'nourishes' the pre-expressive functioning well, the client can (psychologically) benefit and grow from it. 'Growing' in this therapeutic context means that the person, little by little, or sometimes quite suddenly, will take a step forward in reconnecting with reality. From being locked into an idiosyncratic world that may contain delusions, hallucinations, horrifying fears and doubts that function as a kind of fenced prison, to a shift over the 'edge' to become aware again of the not-idiosyncratically distorted, 'objective' or collective reality. This more collective reality is shared by most of us. We are rooted in the everyday and ordinary realities of places, events, things, people, and who are practising socially understandable communication. Explicit awareness of one's own and other's affective functioning is also possible.

Before Prouty, the issue of 'contact' had hardly been the focus of anyone's attention. Rogers (1957) had included it as the first condition of a therapeutic relationship when describing the six necessary and sufficient conditions for constructive personality change. In his work, Prouty (1994; Prouty, Van Werde & Pörtner, 2002) offered a theory and method of how to work with such contact-impaired individuals, opening up the field of person-centred psychotherapy to everyone not previously included and considered as not suited for, or unreachable by, psychotherapy.

In this chapter, we will not only consider the 'difficult edge' represented by the different populations Pre-Therapy has been traditionally applied to, but we will also look at how adjustments and translations can be made in 'classical' Pre-Therapy to meet particular challenges and characteristic ways of being in the world, given extreme positions on the variable of being-in-contact, the so-called 'contact functioning'.

Pre-Therapy and its inspiration for broader contact work

We can distinguish, 'classical' Pre-Therapy (the systematic and intensive use of the contact reflections), from Pre-Therapy translated 'upwards' to dealing with 'grey-zone functioning' and reflections used in working with sudden loss of contact. On a still higher level of contact functioning, we can talk about the idea of 'contact work' as inspiration for how to strengthen newly recovered contact functioning. Translated 'downwards', we can talk about Pre-Therapy developed into concrete ways of being with functioning as encountered in forms of dementia or dying (see Chapter 9). Publications can be found on each of these translations, (see Table 1 for some examples).

Table 1

Levels of contact functioning

Level of contact functioning	Author	Working how, resulting in what
Expressive	Van Werde, 1989	All forms of exercising anchoring, to strengthen freshly regained contact functioning
Sudden loss of contact as in crises or when dissociating	Coffeng, 2005	If needed, one shifts down to 'mere' reflecting, to repair contact that got lost in these specific moments
Grey-zone functioning	Van Werde & Prouty, 2013; Sommerbeck, 2007	Through an apt mix of Pre-Therapy (PT) reflections and 'usual' interventions, first, contact is established, and then, further working together can occur

Pre-expressive functioning	Prouty, 1994	Contact is established due to systematic and intensive use of PT reflecting
Dementia	Dodds, 2008	Episodes of lucidity are fostered with the help of the concrete PT reflections
Dying	Van Werde, 2002	PT reflections as excellent tools for a 'being with' to become a 'letting go'

In this chapter, two examples of Pre-Therapy at difficult edges are presented, one describing being with a dying person, and one about the weekly ward meeting in residential care for people with psychosis. The former touches very low levels of functioning and explores more of a way of letting go, with death in the background; the latter example has contact as an underlying, organising principle of a weekly group meeting, and concerns strengthening the newly recovered but still fragile contact functioning.

Pre-Therapy and being with a dying person

The following vignette (Prouty, 2001, pp. 83–6, taken from Van Werde & Morton, 1999) is a description of a son, familiar with Pre-Therapy and using it to be close to his mother who is lying in a hospital bed and dying of a brain tumour. His intent was not to leave her alone in her dying. So, there is not even a conception of doing psychotherapy – just of compassionate contact.

The five kinds of reflections systematically used in classical Pre-Therapy, aimed at offering contact to people with low levels of contact functioning, are illustrated in this example:

1. SR: *Situational Reflection* reflects the client's situation, environment or milieu. People, places, events and things are reflected to facilitate reality contact. For example, 'a wooden chair', 'the sun is shining in', 'David is entering the room'.

2. FR: *Facial Reflection* reflects pre-expressive feeling embodied in the face to facilitate affective contact, for instance, 'your eyes are wet', 'Hilda smiles'.

3. BR: *Body Reflection* reflects with words or through mimicking with the therapist's or caregiver's own body – or with a combination of both – the movements or positioning of the client. It helps clients to integrate body expression within the sense of self, for example, 'you

point with your finger', or copying the client's action of pointing, or combining the two ways.

4. WWR: *Word-for-Word Reflection* reflects single words, sentence fragments and other possibly disorganised verbal utterances to develop communicative contact, for example, '(mumble), wood, (mumble), three, (mumble)', the therapist reflects 'wood, three', even if the meaning is not clear.

5. RR: *Reiterative Reflection* repeats previous reflections that proved to make contact. It helps to re-establish contact with the client.

These contact reflections (what the therapist does) facilitate the contact functions (client's process) which results in the emergence of contact behaviours (which can be measured). Once overall contact is (re-)established, people can shift to more classical psychotherapy or enjoy the restored contact as it is and profit from the possibilities this holds.[1]

The contact reflections are very well suited to being with someone in a person-centred way, however low the level of functioning may be or – as in the example below – may become. Unlike during most psychotherapy, at these 'edges' of application, no (permanent) shift to higher levels can be expected. Nevertheless, in the following case we will see how, at certain moments, a peak in contact functioning is fostered, with the mother suddenly expressing the first name of her son, followed by the first name and the family name.

> Son: (SR) Now I am sitting on this side of the bed …
>
> (SR) There is more light here …
>
> (SR) I can read better here …
>
> …
>
> (SR) I'm writing a bit …
>
> …
>
> (BR) You hold your hands to your head …
>
> Mother: I was going to read …
>
> Son: (WWR) You were going to read …
>
> Mother: Another paper …
>
> Son: (WWR) Another paper …
>
> Mother: Kellogs? Or what is the name …
>
> Son: [ordinary response] Maalox [a medication]?
>
> Mother: Yes. What?
>
> Son: (WWR) What …

---

1. These possibilities are manifold: from adjusting palliative medication, attending to everyday needs such as eating, drinking and toileting, to enjoying loving human contact.

Mother: What ...

Son: (WWR) What ...

Mother: And which do you have to take then?

Son: (WWR) And which to take ...

    (BR) You keep your hands to your head ...

Mother: Yes.

    ...

Son: (FR) ... and you yawn ...

Mother: Yes, but I have to yawn ...

Son: (WWR) Yes I have to yawn ...

Mother: [yawn, yawn]

Son: (WWR) Yawn ...

Mother: Yes, Kellogs ...

Son: Kellogs ...

Mother: Yes, The Kellogs Book. Yes.

Son: (WWR) Yes ...

    (RR) I came to sit on this side of the bed .... You were talking ...

    ... and your hand was on your head ...

Mother: And that was it.

Son: (WWR) That was it.

Mother: That was it the deliberation

Son: (WWR) The deliberation

    ...

Son: (FR) and you cough ...

Mother: Yes, a bad cough ... I don't like it a bit.

Son: (RR) You cough and say: I don't like it.

Mother: I like it. I don't like it.

    Praying.

Son: (WWR) Praying.

    I like it, I don't like it.

    (RR) and you say 'praying' ...

Mother: Now I am happy.

    Where I'm not happy, I am not happy ...

    And now I am happy.

Son: (WWR) Now you are happy.

Mother: Yes, that is fine, isn't it?

Son: (WWR) That's fine.

Mother: Voilà, that is the way it is. Am I happy, am I happy

    Am I not happy, am I not happy? That's it.

Son: (WWR) That's it.

(RR) You cough and you said: That's it.

Mother: And I cough and cough and cough ...

Son: (WWR) And you say: I cough

(FR, RR) A big yawn and you say I cough.

...

...

(SR) And you are silent now.

Mother: Yes.

...

Three times I do good.

Son: (WWR) Three times I do good.

Mother: Mhm, mhm

[Mother wipes her hands over the sheets.]

Son: (BR) You wipe your hand.

Mother: My hand wipes the little chair.

Son: (WWR) Your hand wipes the little chair.

Mother: I wiped the chair ...

Then I wipe loose ...

Then I don't wipe loose.

Son: (RR) You wiped the chair.

Mother: Then I wipe it loose.

Son: (SR) Your hand is on the pillow.

Mother: It looks like it doesn't it ...

Son: (WWR) It looks like it doesn't it.

Mother: Does somebody finally help me?

Son: (WWR) Does somebody finally help me?

Mother: Do I get help? Yes, don't I?

Son: You ask if you are getting help.

Mother: Yes, It is good. Isn't it?

Son: (WWR) You say it is good.

Mother: It is ... ... [unclear]

Son: (WWR) It is of the boys?

Mother: Grandiose.

Son: (RR, WWR) I hear of the boys and you say grandiose.

Mother: That's what I also heard in the beginning and it isn't true.

Son: (RR) Grandiose.

Mother: Why isn't that OK?

Son: (WWR) Why isn't that OK?

Mother: It is good. Yes.

...

Mother: What is there left to do?

Son: (WWR, BR) What is there left to do? And you hold your hand to your
head.

Mother: What is there still left over then? I want to do something about it
though.

Son: (WWR) I want to do something about it though.

Mother: But what?

Muscles. If all that is good for us. Goody, goody, good.

Son: (WWR, RR) Goody, goody, good. What is still left over?

Mother: If there still is something left over ... You know what I mean 'S'.

Son: (WWR) [surprised and very touched] 'You say my Christian name 'S'.

Mother: 'S' I say 'SQ' [Forename and family name].

Son: (WWR) 'SQ' that's my name.

Mother: That's your name. That's a beautiful name.

Son: [Sits closer and caresses the hand of his mother.]

...

...

(SR) And it turned a little bit darker outside.

Mother: ... and more quiet.

Son: (WWR) [Agreeing and confirming] ... More quiet.

Mother: ... and more quiet that pleases me.

Son: (WWR) And more quiet, that pleases you.

...

[Quiet]

'Contact' as an organising concept for weekly ward meetings in residential care

In many residential care settings the staff organise meetings with patients.
However, the framework and goals of such enterprises are often not clearly
defined. Most of the time, such meetings are about day-to-day issues, the lamps
that need to be repaired or the quality of the food. Such meetings get boring for
staff and patients alike and come to be seen as a necessary evil.

Our strategy was to make the goals explicit and define what belongs in such
a meeting, what does not and why (see also Van Werde in Prouty, Van Werde
& Pörtner, 2002, pp. 61–120). In addition to occasional contact *restoring* work
– when overt psychotic functioning is presented and responded to using Pre-
Therapy reflections – contact *strengthening* became a focus regarding how the
meeting was conceived. This aim is not a luxury, given that everybody on the
ward has had a psychotic episode or is still experiencing one. In relation to the
fields of contact specified by Prouty following Merleau-Ponty (1962), the concept

of the weekly ward meetings then focuses around strengthening communicative contact and contact with reality. In the affective area, anchoring work (helping people to reconnect, to be conscious again, to get 'rooted' within themselves again) can also be done on a group level. This is a unique translation of Pre-Therapy thinking and practice.

The ward meetings take place each Tuesday from 11.10 to 11.50 a.m. with all patients invited, the available nursing staff and the ward psychologist (the author) present. We come together in the living/day room. The day before, during the briefing with nurses, we review the record of the previous meeting. We check to see if points were properly followed up and assemble an informal agenda for the next meeting, for example, introducing a less cumbersome way to organise the meals at noon, announcing the arrival of new patients and so on. In addition to the 'business' aspect of the meeting, attention is also given to how the group as a whole is functioning, which of the patients is having a difficult time and so on. If needed, the staff decides who is going to do some individual contact work in the morning before the meeting with a client suffering a psychotic episode, or who is going to sit next to them for support during the meeting if needed. On very rare occasions we might have to decide to ask someone not to attend because it is felt that it might be too hard on them, on their fellow patients and on the staff if they attended.

The meeting starts with a short introduction about the goal and the ground rules of the meeting. 'It is Tuesday morning, ten past eleven on April the 10th. It is the same every week, we are here together for our ward meeting until about noon. This is so we can have a group conversation. This is not easy, since we are all different. Some find it difficult to talk; others talk too much; for others even sitting here or concentrating is hard work. We want to talk about topics that might possibly be of interest to everybody. Things that are intimate or private belong in a one-to-one conversation with one of the nurses, with me or with your psychiatrist. So, who has a topic to talk about, a comment or a question …?'

If the staff has things to announce or to discuss, this is done at the time in the meeting that seems best suited. We strive for an appropriate balance between concreteness and abstraction, and between open and prepared points for the agenda, to give enough security and trust for people to attend and try to create, for the whole enterprise, a welcoming and anchoring atmosphere.

Strengthening communicative contact

As mentioned earlier, at the beginning of the meeting we explicitly say that we consider the gathering to be a communication exercise. It is not possible to sit together for 45 minutes with such a heterogeneous group of people if the value of the fact of 'mere' talking isn't appreciated. So topics such as the weather, traffic jams, music, how many eggs one is allowed to eat a week and so on are not regarded as trivial or a burden. It is essential to understand that it is therapeutically valuable that someone can be attentive (in a group setting!) for 45 minutes, and can practise this week after week.

The group members don't easily talk spontaneously. We have found that, in order to stimulate communication, a lot of subjects to talk about with a varying of degree of abstraction are required. Very concrete topics probably appeal more to people who are still very much 'locked in' in their world. More abstract themes, a discussion or mere information, are probably more suited for people who function on a higher level. The meeting is neither a mere skill training group nor a psychotherapy group. It is a mixture of both since, besides being task oriented there is always space to talk about anything, be it emotional or interactional. Naturally, group dynamics play a role and can sometimes be intense, which means that careful consideration of who should facilitate the group is crucial.

It is best that the group follows what occupies and interests the participants most at any particular time. When a Scottish historian visited us, we thought that there would be enough to talk about. In fact, only starting from the very concrete here and now of the Scottish plaid skirt of one of the patients could get a conversation going. Other themes were psychologically too distant, too remote from everyday reality.

Another thing we have learned is that there is only conversation in the group as long as something has actually happened on the ward – if people participated or at least felt involved in ward life and daily events. Emptiness – their own as well as that of ward life – can dominate present experience. We have discovered that subjects in which particular patients or staff members have a special interest do very well, for example, to have a conversation about the closing down of the Flemish coal mines when someone from the region of Limburg – a former coal area – shares their experience of losing his job. A German visitor from Heidelberg was directly engaged in conversation by one of the patients who used to be a professional printer and knew that Heidelberg was a brand name of world-famous printing presses.

Reality-oriented work

During each meeting a lot of attention is paid to offering themes about reality. For example, we might mention at the start of each meeting if someone new is expected on the ward, or that there are construction works going on nearby causing traffic jams and delay for visitors and so on. Sometimes we use a playful way to offer and strengthen contact with reality. For example, we might ask what flowers the bouquet on the table is composed of; when the sun rose today (to verify the day-by-day calendar on the wall), how heavy the pumpkin Group II grew in the garden is, and so on. We also bring information from 'outside' inside – something from the newspaper (e.g., a man-made vehicle on Mars), from the radio (e.g., the troubles in Korea) or from staff journeys to work (e.g., sheet ice on the road).

Often the house rules are repeated or refreshed as a follow-up to something that recently went wrong or in connection to a certain atmosphere, for example, 'nobody is allowed in another person's room', or 'no nightwear in the living room'. We also make a big effort to anchor events in time. We try to emphasise any differences between the current meeting, the last and the next meetings. For example, sometimes someone might be quoted from a previous meeting ('You proposed to rent a movie, Paul ...'), or we continue with topics from the last meeting ('You said that you would call the museum to know the opening hours and the rate for groups, Peter ... did you?').

Working on affective contact

We are convinced that a lot of people suffering psychotic functioning aren't always fully aware that they also experience some reality-based, appropriate affects. By the group facilitator actively picking up themes with an affective undertone and by naming this in the group meeting, people can check within themselves if they recognise something congruent with their internal experience. This in itself is therapeutic. Feelings are contacted and acknowledged.

Many themes are cyclic and have an affective load, such as 'saying goodbye', 'being admitted to a hospital', 'being on medication'. Themes like 'emptiness', 'dependence', 'passivity' are always indirectly present in the meeting but are not easily brought to the table. It is important to be cautious and respectful when such themes come to the surface since they are often too confronting and anxiety-provoking, and participants would be frightened away.

If a certain topic is addressed, we always try to hold its reality, communicative and affective aspects in mind. The latter rarely emerge spontaneously, but if they do, they often come very unexpectedly. So, for example, someone can run into his fear of emptiness through a conversation about organising a TV-free evening on the ward, or someone can discover her anxiety about being alone with her husband when hearing somebody announce his discharge from the hospital and looking forward to returning home happily. Frequently, only after systematically reviewing the week does it become evident that a lot must have happened on an emotional level. For example, in one week, two new nurses started on the ward, in addition to occupational and movement therapy students as part of a mental health project. In the ward meeting, we reminded people of all these changes to the day-to-day ward realities and made space for what this might mean emotionally. We asked if anyone remembered any or all of the changes that happened and owned that we had, ourselves, found it a busy week with the influx of lot of new faces. Finally, we wondered if this had had an effect on any patients too.

So, during these meetings, we limit ourselves to actively making space for emotions to be named without going into them in detail, and without processing them individually. It is not always easy to draw a clear line between these two forms of working with affect. We do not do psychotherapy in the strict sense in these meetings, but we do work to strengthen affective contact. Together with the efforts described to strengthen contact with reality and support communication, the format of the weekly ward meeting is a direct translation of Pre-Therapy – structurally building contact work into the group with people recovering from psychotic experiencing in a residential context.

Conclusion

Recognising edges is important, they help definition.

Two translations of Prouty's Pre-Therapy have been described – Pre-Therapy serving two rather extreme edges of contact-impaired functioning. In both palliative care (with very low levels of contact functioning) as well as in working with minor contact loss in a group setting (working with relatively higher levels of contact-impaired functioning, also called 'grey-zone functioning'), the idiom of 'contact' can inspire creative and appropriate ways of working.

In both situations, at the very low as well as at the rather higher level of contact-impaired functioning, and seen from a more technical point of view, giving contact reflections as such disappears more and more into the background. When death is imminent, one shifts from reflecting to a non-verbal presence, whereas when working with the high and anchored ways of functioning, one shifts from using reflections to more traditional therapeutic interventions.

References

Coffeng, T (2005) The therapy of dissociation: Its phases and problems. *Person-Centered & Experiential Psychotherapies, 4*, 90–105.

Dodds, P (2008) Pre-Therapy and dementia care. In G Prouty (Ed) *Emerging Developments in Pre-Therapy: A Pre-Therapy reader* (pp. 15–21). Ross-on-Wye: PCCS Books.

Gendlin, ET (1968) The experiential response. In A Hammer (Ed) *Use of Interpretation in Treatment* (pp. 208–28). New York: Grune and Stratton.

Merleau-Ponty, M (1962) *Phenomenology of Perception* (C Smith, Trans). London: Routledge and Kegan Paul. (Original work published 1945)

Prouty, G (1994) *Theoretical Evolutions in Person-Centered/Experiential Therapy. Applications to schizophrenic and retarded psychoses.* New York: Praeger.

Prouty, G (2001) Unconditional positive regard and Pre-Therapy: An exploration. In JD Bozarth & P Wilkins (Eds) *Rogers' Therapeutic Conditions: Evolution, theory and practice. Vol 3: Unconditional Positive Regard* (pp. 76–87). Ross-on-Wye: PCCS Books.

Prouty, G, Van Werde, D & Pörtner, M (2002) *Pre-Therapy: Reaching contact-impaired clients.* Ross-on-Wye: PCCS Books.

Rogers, CR (1957) The necessary and sufficient conditions of therapeutic personality change. *Journal of Consulting Psychology, 21*(2), 95–103.

Sommerbeck, L (2007) In and out of contact: Therapy with people in the 'grey-zone'. In P Sanders (Ed) *The Contact Work Primer* (pp. 49–59). Ross-on-Wye: PCCS Books.

Van Werde, D (1989) Restauratie van het psychologisch contact bij acute psychose: Een toepassing van Prouty's Pre-Therapy. *Tijdschrift voor Psychotherapie, 15*(5), 271–79.

Van Werde, D (2002) Prouty's Pre-Therapy and contact-work with a broad range of persons' pre-expressive functioning. In G Wyatt & P Sanders (Eds) *Rogers' Therapeutic Conditions: Evolution, theory and practice. Vol 4: Contact and Perception* (pp. 168–81). Ross-on-Wye: PCCS Books.

Van Werde, D & Morton, I (1999) The relevance of Prouty's Pre-Therapy to dementia care. In I Morton (Ed) *Person-Centered Approaches to Dementia Care* (pp. 139–66). Bicester: Winslow Press.

Van Werde, D & Prouty, G (2013) Clients with contact-impaired functioning: Pre-Therapy. In M Cooper, M O'Hara, PF Schmid, & A Bohart (Eds) *The Handbook of Person-Centred Psychotherapy and Counselling* (2nd ed, pp. 327–42). Basingstoke: Palgrave.

Combining person-centred therapy and Pre-Therapy with clients at the difficult edge

6

Lisbeth Sommerbeck

Dion Van Werde (2005) has coined the term 'grey zone' for the many cases concerning people diagnosed with some kind of psychosis or other contact-impairing condition when the counsellor has the experience of being intermittently in good, mutual contact with the client and, at other times, having no clue whatsoever about what is going on in the client. In the latter case, the counsellor can often feel that they might as well be a fly on the wall or that the client has no wish to communicate anything to the counsellor or has no wish to be understood by the counsellor. The client may be expressing something, but it seems inconsequential to the client whether the counsellor is attending to their expressions or not, and even more inconsequential that the counsellor understands their expressions. When the counsellor feels 'out of contact' with a client, the client either seems unable to, or uninterested in, making him- or herself understood to the counsellor or may seem, mistakenly, to take such understanding for granted.

Therefore, in work with people in the grey zone, the counsellor must fluctuate between the ordinary empathic reflectivity of person-centred therapy and the contact reflectivity of Pre-Therapy, depending on whether they believe they are in psychological contact with the client or not.[1] In the first case, the empathic reflectivity of person-centred therapy is appropriate; in the latter case the contact reflectivity of Pre-Therapy is appropriate.

Some grey-zone clients in institutional settings know what psychotherapy is about, ask for it and are able to keep appointments at the therapist's office.[2] For other institutionalised grey-zone clients this is not so, and in these cases it

1. With 'psychological contact' in this context I am thinking of contact where it is possible for the participants to experience the inner frame of reference of the others, i.e., to empathically understand each other.
2. These grey-zone clients may also live on their own and turn up in private practices, in university clinics and the like.

This chapter is adapted from Sommerbeck, L (2007) In and out of contact: Therapy with people in the 'grey-zone'. In P Sanders (Ed) *The Contact Work Primer* (pp. 49–60). Ross-on-Wye: PCCS Books.

is the therapist's desire to contact the client that fuels the relationship in what can sometimes be a very long beginning phase. This means that the therapist makes a purely unilateral decision to try to actively make contact with a client at regular times and places that have the best chance of finding the client receptive and open to contact. Later, though, if the client is responding to the contact with the therapist, they may eagerly be waiting for the therapist at the normal set time for the therapy session. Even so, it can be a long time before the client is able to, or interested in, making and keeping an agreement to meet with the therapist in the consulting room at pre-scheduled times. Relationships with some of the more disturbed grey-zone clients may never develop that far, yet despite this, such efforts by the therapist may still contribute to improving the quality of life of the client by enabling them to share more of their life and experiences with others.

What follows are two examples (to protect confidentiality any identifying content has been changed) of individual psychotherapeutic contact in the grey zone.[3] One is with a client who was motivated for psychotherapy from her own volition. The other is with a client for whom the idea of psychotherapy was apparently far beyond his grasp, and so it was the therapist who initiated and upheld the contact. In both examples, situational reflections, bodily reflections, word-for-word reflections, facial reflections, iterative reflections and empathic reflections are marked SR, BR, WWR, FR, IR and ER, respectively. The therapist follows no rules in responding with one or the other kind of reflection, only her sense of what is in the moment-to-moment focus of the client's attention.

Lillian

Lillian is diagnosed with paranoid schizophrenia. She is, however, functioning well enough to be actively motivated for psychotherapy and to be able to make and keep appointments, so she comes to the therapist's office for pre-scheduled talks. In their first three sessions she talks rather freely of her conviction that her new neighbours are out to kill her and even if the content of her narrative is a paranoid delusion, she reveals much of what is going on in her with respect to this particular conception of reality and the therapist is therefore able to respond almost exclusively with empathic reflections. In the fourth session, however, her condition has changed; all energy seems drained out of her, she sits with her head bent down so the therapist cannot see her face, and she does not start talking from her own initiative as she has done in previous sessions. She sits like this for some minutes, and the therapist has no idea of what is going on in her.

---

3. These examples first appeared in Sommerbeck, L (2003) *The Client-Centred Therapist in Psychiatric Contexts: A therapists' guide to the psychiatric landscape and its inhabitants*. Ross-on-Wye: PCCS Books.

T0:   We sit in silence and you have bent your head down. (SR, BR)

L1:   [L stays in the same position for a while. Then she raises her head a little and takes both her hands to her head, pulling her hair and using her hair as 'handles' to shake her head.]

T1:   [Mirroring her gesture.] You shake your head with your hair. (BR)

L2:   [L lets her hands sink into her lap and turns to look at the therapist with what seems like an expression of hopelessness in her face and eyes.]

T2:   You look hopeless? (FR)

L3:   [Looking down again.] Yes ... I don't know.

T3:   You said: 'Yes', and 'I don't know'. (WWR)

L4:   I don't know what to say – I'm so tired.

T4:   Too tired even to talk, is that how you feel? (ER)

L5:   Yes ... yes.
       [There is a long pause, where T stays silent and L remains motionless, with her head bent down, as in the start of the session. Then the loud 'cock-a-doodle-doo!' of a nearby cockerel is heard and L raises her head and looks towards the window.]

T5:   You look up at the sound of the cockerel. (BR, SR)

L6:   [Turns towards the therapist and smiles, and the therapist smiles back at her.]

T6:   You looked up at the sound of the cock and now we smile at each other, and you look glad. (RR, SR, FR)

L7:   We used to have lots of animals at home when I was a kid; cocks, too; sometimes they kept everybody awake [giggles].

T7:   [Smiling.] Feels good and funny, recalling that, right? (ER)

L8:   Yes [looking sad], I wish I could be there again.

T8:   You look sad when you think of how you miss being at home as a kid. (FR, ER)

L9:   Yes, I wish I had my family, I feel so lonely, and I don't know what to do, I'm scared of returning home.

T9:   'If I had a family to return home to, I wouldn't feel so lonely and scared', is that it? (ER)

L10: Yes, K [her primary nurse] proposed the other day that I try to go home to my apartment with her, one of these days, to see how it feels; I think they want me to go home soon.

T10: You think they see you as being ready to go home soon, but you don't feel ready at all. You feel they hurry you a bit? (ER)

L11: Yes, but I think I should try to go home with K.

T11: You feel you ought to give it a try? (ER)

L12: Yes, I really don't know what to do, how I shall manage at home. I'm not so scared of the neighbours anymore, but still, maybe I'll do something that disturbs them, so they'll complain about me to the janitor and have me thrown out of the apartment, that's what I'm thinking about all the time.

T12: You just worry so much that you won't do things right at home, that you'll somehow displease your neighbours? (ER)

L13: Maybe – they have two children so they are four and I'm alone, and their apartment is the same size as mine ...

T13: Feels as if you haven't got the right to occupy that much space when they have so little? (ER)

L14: I know I've got the right, of course, but still ... I guess I feel somehow guilty about it ... But that's only ... it's weighing me down, the thoughts; they keep turning and turning around in my head. [Bends her head down and away again, saying this.]

T14: [Again feeling somewhat out of contact with L.] You said 'It's weighing me down' and you bend your head. (WWR of the part of the client's statement that seemed most meaningful to her, combined with BR.)

L15: [After a long pause, almost inaudible.] I don't think I can go home with K, do you think she will be annoyed with me?

T15: I don't know, I wish I could tell you for sure that she wouldn't be, 'cause I guess you are really afraid to displease her? (Answer to L's question, ER.)

L16: Yes, she has done a lot for me and she offers to escort me home, and then I can't even think of trying.

T16: Like there'd be nothing you'd wish more than to feel able to accept her offer and feel helped by it, but instead you feel burdened by it, is it something like that? (ER)

L17: Yes, very, and I don't know how to tell her.

From this point the therapist had, again, a steady sense of mutuality in the contact with Lillian, and the therapist could thus receive Lillian's continuing considerations of how she'd deal with K's offer with the ordinary empathic reflectivity of client-centred therapy. In this case, K's idea of escorting Lillian on a home visit had stimulated a kind of crisis reaction in Lillian by which she lost some of her normally good contact functioning. Being received, in this phase, with pre-therapeutic contact reflections helped Lillian back to her ordinary level of relatively good mutual contact with others. In particular, Lillian regained her normally enjoyable contact with K with whom she managed to make a deal about home visits that was satisfactory to both parties.

Svend

Svend is also diagnosed with paranoid schizophrenia. He is, however, not nearly as well-functioning, with respect to contact, as Lillian. He rarely seeks contact with others; there seems to be nothing he wants others to understand about himself and he expresses no need for help, psychotherapy or otherwise. He was not involuntarily admitted to the psychiatric hospital, but let himself, passively, be taken in. The wish to enter into a psychotherapeutic relationship is not the client's wish; it is the therapist's wish, so the therapist is the one who takes the initiative to talk with Svend in his room on the ward. This excerpt is from the sixth session. After Svend has declared his willingness to talk with the therapist, the therapist clears a stack of clothes from a chair and sits down.

T0: I thought that maybe ... if there was anything you might like to tell me today, about how you feel, and about your situation, how you look on it?

C1: [In a very matter of fact, 'there's no discussing it', way.] I feel well.

T1: You say you feel well, and you look very determinedly at me. (WWR, FR)

C2: Yes, I feel well, and that's a fact.
[Pause, C looks down at his lap.]

T2: You say it's a fact you feel well, and now you look down and are quiet. (WWR, BR)

C3: Yes, I feel well when I drink coffee, juice, and things like that, but water is no good – and I've stopped eating.

T3: As long as you can drink something that tastes good you feel well, but you've lost your appetite? (ER)

C4: Yes, and I also feel well because I'm now totally out of the church.

T4: It's a relief to be finally out of it. (ER)

C5: Yes, well, I'm not totally out of it, I still receive their newsletter, and I can't read it, it was a mistake that I joined the church, I'm confused about it – I have to tell them to stop sending the newsletter.

T5: The church was really too much, and now you need to get that newsletter off your back, that'll be a relief? (ER)

C6: Yes, that's it, I need to stop the newsletter and to have my mail delivered here, then I can feel fine – but I do feel fine here.

T6: You like to be here, and if you had these things settled you could enjoy it better, be more at ease? (ER)

C7: Yes, precisely, that would be nice.
[Pause. C moves his head around in abrupt jerks, staring at different spots.]

T7: You turn your head this way and that way and look around. (BR)

C8: [Grinding his teeth.] My father is Satan.

T8: You grind your teeth and say 'My father is Satan'. (FR, WWR)

C9: He has slaughtered my mother, he is the real Satan, and the Danes are his devils and devils' brood.

T9: He is the real Satan, because he has slaughtered your mother, and the Danes are his devils and devils' brood. (WWR)

C10: Not all Danes, people here are nice to me, but he has slaughtered my mother and if he does it again I'll slaughter him.

T10: You feel you'll slaughter him if ... (WWR)

[C interrupts eagerly and vehemently with his voice raising.]

C11: Yes, he has terrorised my mother all her life, psychological terror … her name is Maria, if Satan harmed Maria … Joseph would slaughter him, I'm Joseph.

T11: You say 'I'm Joseph' and you feel like you think Joseph would feel if Satan harmed Maria, is that it? (WWR, ER)

C12: [Nodding his head and smiling.] Yes, and I'm not afraid of Satan, I'm not afraid of anything.

T12: You smile at the thought that you are not afraid of Satan or … (FR, WWR)

C13: [Interrupting.] Yes, I'm not afraid, I'm glad of that, but why does he always have to be so rotten, last time he visited he brought some fruit from his back garden; it smelled awful and then I took a bite and it tasted hellish … I threw it all away.

T13: You think that everything he brings … (ER?)

C14: [Interrupting.] Yes, why does he have to be so provocative?

T14: Like 'Why the hell can't you buy me some good fruit that I like, instead of bringing me the rotten leftovers from your back garden?' (ER)

C15: Yes, I think he never spreads anything but shit around him – I can't bear being near him.

The client spends the rest of the session exploring his relationship with his father in a way that seems much more coherent and less infiltrated with psychotic ideation than in the first part of the session and in a way that makes empathic reflections more appropriate than contact reflections. When the client and the therapist take leave of each other Svend heads towards the nurses' office to secure their help with resigning his membership of the rather fundamentalist religious sect of which he has been a member. Thus, during the session his reality function, in particular, improved. It should be noted, however, that such improvement is rarely lasting with clients like Svend. Ordinarily, the next session will start on more or less the same level of contact functioning as the previous one and improvement is at best a '2 steps forward, 1.9 steps back' process. More steady improvement takes a very long time (ordinarily years), so it is a sine qua non that the therapist has the capacity of patience and still more patience. However, no matter how patient the therapist is, it is the rare therapist who will not sometimes despair, lose confidence in themselves, and fail to see the often very subtle signs of progress. It is therefore important that the therapist has access to a support group that understands what they are trying to accomplish.

In the transcribed session with Svend, it is characteristic that he jumps from one issue to the next without the therapist seeing any connection between the issues of feeling well, his drinking habits, the church and his father. This is characteristic of work with clients like Svend, with whom the therapist must tolerate that there often seems to be no 'red thread' joining the issues the client touches upon. It's important that the therapist does not hold on to a particular issue in order to satisfy their own wish for coherence and understanding of the connection between one issue and the next.

The reader might also note therapist response T11. This is really a bad response, clumsy, long-winded and too abstract. The reason was the therapist's momentary loss of full concentration on the client's perspective. A mental picture of the client killing his father disturbed the therapist's concentration and had her momentarily scared and thus, in her response, she distanced herself from the full intensity and vehemence of the client's statement. Perhaps C12 shows that the client picked up the therapist's feeling of fear. A much better response would have been: 'I'm Joseph, I'll slaughter him if he harms Maria', stated with some of the client's intensity. However, the therapist regains her full concentration in the following responses, and the bad response doesn't seem to influence the client's progression to better reality contact toward the end of the session. Therapists are fallible, and if their failures are the exception rather than the rule, they normally do not influence the process in any significantly negative way.

Reference

Van Werde, D (2005) Facing psychotic functioning: Person-centred contact work in residential psychiatric care. In S Joseph & R Worsley (Eds) *Person-Centred Psychopathology: A positive psychology of mental health* (pp. 158–68). Ross-on-Wye: PCCS Books.

A person-centred approach to counselling clients with autistic process

7

Anja Rutten

Publications about people with autism tend to use medical language, with terms like *disorder, abnormal* and *symptoms*. My perspective on autistic process rejects medicalisation, and in this chapter, I will use the terms *autism* and *autistic process* to describe people who experience themselves, others and the world in ways that are not *neurotypical* (the term for 'not autistic') or conforming to the norm.

One of the major features that distinguishes person-centred theory from other approaches is its reluctance or refusal to conceptualise human distress in medical terms (Sanders, 2013). There have been helpful theoretical conceptualisations in person-centred theory that take account of clients whose style of processing the world is not typical, and that use non-stigmatising language. Some examples of these processes are psychotic process (Prouty, Van Werde & Pörtner, 2002) and fragile and dissociated processes (Warner, 2005, 2007, see also Chapter 10 by Margaret Warner in this volume). These concepts have been useful in allowing counsellors to talk about particular subgroups of clients without the need to borrow medical terminology and take on the underlying, irreconcilable, principles of the medical model. For this reason I suggest that *autistic process* needs to be added to the processes above as a distinct process.

Autistic process is a minority process. It is not pathological, nor a sign of mental ill health, but it *is* different. A consequence of autistic process is that, compared with neurotypical people, there are *qualitative* differences in how people view and make sense of the world. The effects of living with autism can be profound and pervasive.

The social model of disability views disability as largely arising from society's attitudes towards difference (Oliver, 1990, 1996) and this is clearly demonstrated in the experience of people with autistic process. Common difficulties imposed by society and experienced by people with autism are very often the logical outcome of non-acceptance of different processing styles. High levels of unpredictability in day-to-day life clash with a great need for predictability; difficulties shifting attention in a fast-paced ever-changing environment set people apart and put them at risk of social rejection and isolation. The stress and anxiety resulting from these experiences can be overwhelming. As a cautionary note, whilst counselling can help make sense of and come to terms with negative experiences, people with autistic process often face discrimination and exclusion. It would be a mistake to see counselling as the answer if this is society's only response to distress caused by social injustice.

This chapter will focus mainly on people with autistic process who are willing and able to engage in counselling. It will start with describing some of the common areas in which people with autism experience difficulties or differences. The second part of the chapter will focus on person-centred work.

Introduction to autism

The National Autistic Society defines autism as '… a lifelong developmental disability that affects how a person communicates with, and relates to, other people. It also affects how they make sense of the world around them' (www.autism.org.uk). All people with autistic process experience difficulties in their communication (both verbal and non-verbal), social interaction and relationships with others and use of social imagination (including seeing things from other people's perspectives). In addition, people with autism often have sensory difficulties and a narrow or restricted range of interests. Autism is usually detectable by age 3 (albeit often retrospectively). It is pervasive, that is, it manifests across social settings and affects multiple aspects of life. In the literature this combination of affected areas of social functioning is often referred to as the *triad of impairments* (Wing, 1996).

What causes autism is unknown, although it is highly probable that a variety of genes are involved in its aetiology, potentially in conjunction with various environmental triggers. The current ratio of four men to every woman may support a genetic explanation, although some query whether autism simply presents differently (and is recognised less easily) in women (National Institute for Health and Care Excellence (NICE), 2011).

Autism is commonly thought of as falling along a spectrum of intellectual ability, with approximately 25 per cent (Bowler, 2007) to 50 per cent (NICE, 2011) of people on that spectrum defined as learning disabled (IQ < 70). The term 'autism' tends to be used to describe the whole of the spectrum as well as the learning disabled end of the spectrum (which is also referred to as Kanner's autism), whilst Asperger syndrome, Asperger's Disorder and High-Functioning Autism are exclusively used for those people who are not considered to have a learning disability. The terms 'Autism Spectrum Disorder' and 'Autism Spectrum Condition' describe the whole spectrum. The term 'Pervasive Developmental Disorder Not Otherwise Specified' (PDD-NOS) captures autism that does not neatly fall into the other specified categories (*Diagnostic and Statistical Manual of Mental Disorders*, 4th ed., text rev., *DSM-IV-TR*).

The arrival of *Diagnostic and Statistical Manual of Mental Disorders, 5th edition* (*DSM-5*) heralded the introduction of the term 'Autism Spectrum Disorder' for all people on the spectrum and does away with different 'labels'. In this version, indications of severity in several subsections, rather than intellectual ability, determine someone's degree of autism. A discussion of the advantages and disadvantages of labelling people with autistic process in this way falls outside of the scope of this chapter, but this subject has generated a lot of debate, and affects in particular those people with autism who define themselves (and were previously diagnosed) as having Asperger syndrome.

Living with autistic process

People with autistic process live in this world as a minority, making up about 1 per cent of the population (NICE, 2011). The effects of living with autism can be profound and affect multiple areas of experiencing and processing. People with autism have a differently abled way of being in the world, but often, in addition to this, encounter problems that arise from not being accepted, which can become disabling (Bauminger, Shulman & Agam, 2003; Kelly, Garnett, Attwood & Peterson, 2008; White & Roberson-Nay, 2009). Natasha (all names and identifying details have been changed), in one of her counselling sessions with me, described it like this: 'It's the signals that I give off as an autistic person, somehow being different and to others I give off, like a red flag, and then people can be rude to me and that's stressing me.'

Having thought about her encounters with others in counselling, Natasha has come to the conclusion: 'I love being me and I love my autism. I am honest, I don't compromise on my principles. I can't see why that is a problem to other people. They tell me it is, but I was fed up with trying to please them and always failing, so I have given up trying to fit in, and I am just me now.'

People describe living with autistic process both in terms of challenges and advantages. For example, John, another client, talks about his difficulties in having to cope with too many social stimuli and insufficient time to process them: 'At the moment, I'm not working but when I was working, it was constant stress and trying to cope with other people, trying to keep up with working amongst other people. Not having time to process the information throughout the day led to very poor mental health.' He goes on to describe some of his strengths: 'I find working as a web designer solving problems, finding out what had gone wrong in a piece of code, may be easier for me than for some other people.'

People with autism frequently want to begin and maintain relationships and to have social contact with others, but experience difficulties in doing so (Attwood, 2006; Bauminger, 2002). Social interactions are of vital importance for day-to-day functioning and are reliant on unspoken and inconsistent rules and conventions. They require flexibility in thought, emotion and behaviour. Verbal language is only a small proportion of our communication, and pitch, intonation, gestures, facial expressions and body posture all contribute to the messages we transmit. In addition, these conventions are culturally determined and socially constructed. The majority of people with autistic process have problems precisely with these elements.

Josh illustrates this when he talks about his sadness not having found a life partner: 'Every time I like someone, she's either married or not interested in me. I have had a girlfriend, but she left me. She wanted me to go to parties with her, but I wanted to stay at home because it was Friday and I wanted to watch TV like I always do. When I did go to Esther's party with her, she was very angry with me afterwards, and said I should not have talked to Patrick about his life insurance for so long. She says she tried to hint to me that I needed to stop, but I did not know why she was pulling faces at me.'

Many people with autism have difficulties working out or anticipating other people's thoughts, emotions and intentions (and sometimes also their own) and these are key elements of any neurotypical social encounter. In the autism literature these problems are historically seen as outcomes of problems with theory of mind (ToM) (the ability to take others' perspectives) (e.g., Baron-Cohen, 1995; Mitchell, 1997). The closest a neurotypical person could probably get to this experience of those difficulties is imagining being in a culturally alien (and possibly unwelcoming) environment. Ways of interacting with others seem to make sense to everyone else and there is a constant sense of getting it wrong, without clear understanding of, or help in, getting it right.

'Reading' social situations requires shifting of attention and getting the 'gist' of the situation, rather than all the minutiae. Those aspects of experiencing and processing too are often difficult for people with autism, as they tend to prefer a processing style that is detail-focused (Bowler, 2007). The academic literature on executive function (which drives attention shifting) and 'weak' versus 'strong' central coherence (processing detail versus gist) can be accessed through, for example, Bowler (2007).

Recent advances in neuropsychological research indicate that there may be differences in mirror neurones in people with autistic process, and this may lead to differences in empathic functioning and perspective taking (Hamilton, Brindley & Frith, 2007; Jacob, 2008). Practitioners might be more familiar with the concept of 'mentalising' from psychotherapy literature (Allen, Fonagy & Bateman, 2008). Debates in these areas are complex and detailed, but essentially boil down to the fact that social relationships can be severely hampered when someone is not able to work out what someone else might be thinking or feeling. At best this leads to confusion and misunderstandings, but there are also more serious consequences for people with autistic process, such as social vulnerability leading to a higher risk of becoming a victim of crime, violence and abuse (Petersilia, 2001).

The lives of most neurotypical people are reasonably predictable and if unexpected things happen, a range of coping strategies is available to deal with and compensate for lack of certainty and sudden changes. This flexibility to adapt to uncertainty requires a considerable amount of imagination. Generating alternative scenarios in one's mind and choosing strategies to employ in any given situation draws on the ability to be flexible. For people with autistic process these skills are not always easy to develop and use (Baron, Groden, Groden & Lipsitt, 2006). Consequently, people with autism are often stressed about uncertainty. Unexpected changes are not necessarily objectively 'big', but could result from a minor change in routine, such as the bus taking a different route due to roadworks. Support is frequently required to help predict situations or cope with anxiety resulting from uncertainty. Given that other human beings are often far from consistent, people can be a source of comfort because of the support they can offer, as well as a source of distress because of their inconsistency.

In addition to difficulties or differences in communication, interaction and imagination, people with autistic process often have different sensory experiences. They frequently also have a narrow range of interests (APA, 2013; NICE, 2011). Sensory differences can affect all senses, and can manifest as oversensitivity, undersensitivity, or a combination. For example, someone may find bright lights unbearable, but could be unresponsive to loud noise. Routines are often favoured, sometimes to the extent of not being able or willing to change any aspect of this. Of course this is not always detrimental, and for some people, a strong and narrow focus helps build successful careers because of the high level of expertise developed. Others, however, do not fare so well and struggle with daily life.

The way in which autism affects people varies. Some have more difficulties in one area than another, whilst others are having problems and strengths in fairly equal measures. This of course has an effect on how people relate to themselves, others and the world, and this includes how they would use the therapeutic relationship in counselling.

Autistic process and mental health

The descriptions of aspects of autistic process above illustrate that living with autism can be deeply rewarding, but also very stressful. Delayed processing of events and a high level of painful life experiences are common in this client group. People with autism may behave in atypical ways. This sets them apart as 'different', which frequently results in interpersonal problems. Part of the distress experienced by many is the result of being ignored, ridiculed and bullied. Social exclusion and isolation are extremely common. It is well known that good social contacts and networks act as buffers against poor mental health (Segrin, 2001), but people with autism often have few social contacts and small networks.

Research into levels of mental health difficulties in people with autism shows that these are indeed extremely common, with 65 per cent of people with autistic process thought to have mental health difficulties (Deudney & Shah, 2001). In adults, feeling anxious or depressed, obsessive-compulsive behaviours, thoughts and rituals are particularly common (Gillott et al., 2001; Howlin, 1997a, b; Tantam, 2000). Adolescents with high-functioning autism experience significantly more problems with feeling depressed or anxious than their neurotypical peers (Kim et al., 2000). In children, difficulties sustaining attention (often labelled as attention deficit hyperactivity disorder) are also frequent (Ghaziuddin et al., 1998).

Counselling people with autistic process

Most academic publications about successful psychotherapeutic work with clients with autism are based on cognitive-behavioural approaches (e.g., Cardaciotto & Herbert, 2004; Schuurman, 2010) with recent developments in mindfulness-based therapy (Spek, 2010; Spek et al., 2010). A few articles report using different theoretical orientations such as personal construct psychology (Hare, Jones & Paine, 1999) and psychodynamic therapy (e.g., Mero, 2002). A limited number of studies report the outcomes of randomised controlled trials of group therapy using a cognitive-behavioural approach (Sofronoff, Attwood, & Hinton, 2005; Sofronoff, Attwood, Hinton, & Levin, 2007).

Publications from a person-centred perspective are currently few and far between and I do not know of any that are based on outcome research. An article by Carrick and McKenzie (2011) presents a heuristic study of training professionals in the use of Pre-Therapy skills with people who work with clients who have autism and difficulties in making psychological contact. One book chapter discusses a person-centred approach to a psychology service for children with autism (Knibbs & Moran, 2005). An argument has also been made in the Dutch-language literature that autism-specific knowledge for person-centred counsellors can act as a helpful way into the client's world (Stinckens & Becaus, 2008). Recently, Vuijk (2013) described how therapy that is process-oriented and based on person-centred principles can work with clients with autism.

All in all, the current evidence base for therapy with people with autistic process is still in its infancy. Whilst there are reports that various types of counselling are effective for people with high-functioning autism, most studies are from a cognitive-behavioural paradigm, based on very small samples, group-based and often with children who have an IQ within the typical range, or no more than a mild learning disability. They are not representative of the range of people with autism.

In some ways, cognitive-behavioural outcome studies may be good news for clients with autism because the studies raise clients' profile with therapists, although they also emphasise therapist expertise and technique. It should be borne in mind, however, that research (with neurotypical populations) consistently shows that it is not counsellor modality or technique, but client variables, extra-therapeutic factors and the therapeutic relationship that are the main features in accounting for therapy outcomes (Asay & Lambert, 1999). Clients might have preferences for particular styles of counselling and may do better with particular types of counsellors at different times (Cooper & McLeod, 2007). Clients therefore need to be able to access the full range of counselling opportunities, not just the services that 'gatekeepers' allow them access to. This applies to people with autism as much as to the 'average' client – but perhaps more so given the highly idiosyncratic nature of autistic process.

Adults with autism report that they want to access therapeutic relationships and many see value in counselling (personal communications). My conversations with people with autistic process about their needs and experiences of counselling have highlighted that there is a dire need for therapeutic relationships that are relational in nature. Unfortunately it appears that therapy like this is not easily accessible and that, often, therapy experiences are not satisfactory. In addition to lack of choice about type of therapy, adults and parents of children with autism, report they are (illegally) excluded from mainstream mental health services on the basis of their autistic process, thus leaving them without support and help when this is needed.

The anxiety resulting from living as a person with autism can be both traumatising and alienating, and being understood in a safe environment has potential to help clients. In research on successful therapy outcomes, relationship factors have consistently been found to be of great importance (Norcross, 2002) and no significant differences are found between therapy outcomes for different modalities (Cooper, 2008; King et al., 2013), once researcher allegiance effects (the tendency to find supporting evidence for one's own therapy) have been controlled for (Luborsky et al., 1999; Wampold, 2001). The prima facie argument for person-centred therapy is therefore at the very least as strong as for any other therapeutic approach.

Person-centred counselling with clients with autistic process

Clients with autism can present with a wide range of issues, just like neurotypical clients, and it is not the aim of this chapter to provide a 'problem-based' overview of working with this client group. There are, however, some relatively frequent differences which largely revolve around communication and relationship styles, in addition to difficulties with accessing and processing experiences (including feelings and thoughts about experiences) and the tendency not to generalise experience.

Communication and relationships

Person-centred theory describes all living organisms as having an actualising tendency, which is the single drive for growth and differentiation. Communication and relationships are of vital importance to humans and person-centred theory emphasises the pro-social nature of human beings (Rogers, 1951). Our sense of self emerges from our relationships, and significant others have considerable impact on how we see ourselves.

People with autistic process are no exception to this. The impact of socialisation on the formation of their self-concept may, however, be very different from that of neurotypical people. For people with autistic process, whose difficulties are largely in the social domain, life is likely to start off with disadvantages, as the source of connection with and learning from others is also a major source of difficulty. When social interaction and communication are fraught with difficulties, positive experiences are likely to be reduced and this will have an effect on how people feel and think about themselves. It is probable that social interactions with significant others in early life present people with autism with very high levels of conditionality. Whilst conditions of worth and incongruence develop like this in the neurotypical population too, for people with autism there is an additional dimension.

Difficulties with shifting attention, imagination and decreased flexibility may present competing forces: when very embedded in one's own perspective, it is more difficult to take the perspective of someone else and see why social demands and requests, made explicitly or implicitly, may need to be taken into consideration. It is therefore not inconceivable that the development and maintenance of conditions of worth in people with autistic process follow a different trajectory to that of people with neurotypical process, and that the nature of incongruence in autistic process may also differ to that in the neurotypical population.

None of these issues need be problematic for person-centred counsellors. Rogers (1951, p. 494) asserts that 'the best vantage point for understanding behavior is from the internal frame of reference of the individual himself'. Empathic listening will help therapists enter a client's frame of reference just like they would with neurotypical clients. A very high level of precision and accuracy may be required, and this may require a higher level of patience and consistent empathic understanding from the therapist. In many ways though, this process is no different from listening to clients with fragile process or to clients who are out of psychological contact.

In the next example, Amanda talks about what it is like to have autism. She struggles with the idea that it is OK not to be totally accurate in conversations and construes this as 'mistakes'. She notices that her struggle impacts on her relationships with others, but she is unable to adapt her communication style.

> Amanda: If I make a mistake then I worry that people will think 'she's not always that accurate'. I do still make mistakes occasionally, but I usually have an idea that I am, that I'm probably, it's probably not quite right if I'm making a mistake.
>
> George: So you usually know when you make a mistake, that you're not quite right. And it sounds like making mistakes is a big deal for you, because you worry about what other people might think. Is that right?
>
> Amanda: Yeah. I think that other people think that if I make mistakes, then when I know that I'm not making a mistake they might think that I could be making a mistake because usually if I do make a mistake I've got an idea that it's not quite right, but I can't work out at that point what's not right about it. But then sometimes if you try to tell people later that something wasn't right before, they don't think it's important to still be saying something about 'oh I told you this last week, but actually, it was, I meant it like this'. And they're like 'So?'
>
> George: For them it's not very important and in their view it's gone, and you're still working on it because for you it's really important. It's like you're ... what? Out of synch?
>
> Amanda: Yeah and I can never get it right, and my brother doesn't like me because he says I am pedantic and I didn't even mean to be but he was wrong about the time we went on holiday to Llandudno because it was definitely not in September [sighs and tears well up].

Amanda's therapist knows it is very important for her to be accurately understood, especially given the topic of conversation. Amanda's final response indicates that she feels understood, and this allows her to access more detail about a conversation, and some of her feelings, so that they can be experienced more fully.

Experiencing, processing, remembering and generalising

The example above shows another major difference between typical and autistic process. This relates to how events are experienced, processed and stored in long-term memory. Clients with autism frequently experience the world around them in great detail, and this can impede the sharing of narratives, because the 'gist' of stories can be lost (Bowler, 2007). Neurotypical people have choices about the trade-off between detail and main thread. They generally accommodate their listeners fairly automatically, prioritising their need for relating over their need for precision. Clients with autistic process may not be easily able to trade detail for gist, or they may have difficulties in feeling the importance of social and communicative aspects of sharing experience.

People with autism often get overloaded by the amount of incoming information (cognitive, emotional and sensory). In addition to a detail-focused processing style, and a likely backlog of experience that has not been processed, they do not appear to use the same strategies of forgetting or ignoring information. Where neurotypical people 'strip' experience and schematise information to form a very efficient, but not very precise, memory system, people with autism seem to use more linear, serial strategies to store information in episodic memory (Bowler, 2007). This way of storing information lends itself to specificity and accuracy, and there are distinct advantages to that. In some situations (e.g., developing computer code) it is of great importance.

Related to this is that unprocessed issues, sometimes from a long time ago, can come up seemingly out of nowhere and cause great distress. It is also not uncommon for people to have an interest that they like talking about, and sooner or later, their conversations end up with that interest. Clients with autistic process often indicate that letting go of past experiences can be extremely difficult and they may talk repetitively about the same issues, often apparently without resolving them.

In content-directive and expert-led therapies there is some respite for the counsellor, in that they can take charge of the session and steer the client towards what they 'need' to talk about. Person-centred therapists, however, are careful with directing clients and do not take an expert position. There is debate about acceptability of process-guiding, but the general consensus is that content direction is unhelpful (Sanders, 2012).

Some person-centred therapists feel that process guidance assists clients with autistic process make sense of a long line of 'horizontal' and unintegrated experiences. A level of process direction may also help build opportunities for generalising experiences from therapy to other settings and relationships, as generalisation in people with autistic process does not usually happen to the same extent as it does for neurotypical people unless it is fostered (Bowler, 2007).

It is not the case that all experiences are equally important to people with autism, but it can be enormously difficult for clients to see that 'in the moment'. A narrow range of interests and decreased flexibility to change the theme of the conversation can lead to going 'off track' and onto long monologues about a favoured topic. Whilst this may look like the client is avoiding their experience, this may not be the case. It can be difficult to know whether the client is actually intending to talk themselves away from what they were exploring, and clients do not always realise this is what they are doing.

Classically oriented person-centred therapists might favour continuing to follow the client in their experience. This may be of great therapeutic benefit to the client. It is not common to be heard so fully when talking about something that is likely to meet with boredom or attempts to change the topic from others in day-to-day life. Being able to finish talking about something also enables letting go of it.

As a therapist who incorporates process-experiential principles into person-centred work, I generally discuss with clients what they would like me to do when I observe this 'going onto a different track' happening. I may ask them what would best meet their needs and whether this is something that happens because of, or despite, what they want to talk about. I have no investment in staying with the client at that point, or helping them get back to another topic, but aim to offer clients choices about process. This too may be therapeutic, in that it signals to the client that there is space for all of their experience and that their therapeutic needs are taken seriously.

Whatever level of process direction is offered, a good quality therapeutic relationship offering congruence, empathy and unconditional positive regard in high measures remains vitally important, especially because very often relationships with these qualities are woefully absent in the lives of people with autistic process.

Conclusion

To date there are very few opportunities for counsellors (person-centred or otherwise) who want to work with people on the autistic spectrum to gain knowledge and skills in formal training settings, although this is starting to change. In the counselling room, most work (person-centred or otherwise) is undertaken in an ad hoc and idiosyncratic way. Idiosyncrasy is not necessarily bad: the counselling relationship is highly individual to client and counsellor and this is one of the strengths of person-centred work.

However, arising from this status quo is the reality that far too often it is left up to the client with autistic process to educate their counsellor. Counsellors have a professional responsibility to educate themselves about client groups so that our client can help us get to know them personally, rather than getting to know simply about their 'category memberships'. Whilst it is to some extent inevitable that counsellors are introduced to the world of the client and learn about the client through this, we would (or should!) not expect gay clients to educate us on all aspects of being gay, nor would we expect women clients to educate us about the basics of being a woman. Despite the highly individual nature of autism, there are a number of common elements in autistic process, and they might be useful information for counsellors who are looking to work with this group of clients (Stinckens & Becaus, 2008).

As long as person-centred counsellors are able to work from their client's frame of reference and accommodate their client's needs, they need not be worried that somehow it is not possible to work with clients with autism in a person-centred way. In my view it is a myth that counsellors need to do more, direct session content or somehow compensate for their clients' autism. Whilst clients with autism may have a qualitatively different process, there is nothing 'wrong' with that and it does not need 'fixing'. Person-centred approaches offer a genuine relationship that is accepting and empathic and this is a very good basis for working with clients with autistic process.

References

Allen, JG, Fonagy, P & Bateman, AW (2008) *Mentalizing in Clinical Practice*. Washington, DC: American Psychiatric Publishing.

American Psychiatric Association (2000) *Diagnostic and Statistical Manual of Mental Disorders* (4th ed, text rev). Washington, DC: American Psychiatric Association.

American Psychiatric Association (2013) *American Psychiatric Association: Diagnostic and Statistical Manual of Mental Disorders* (5th ed). Arlington, VA: American Psychiatric Association.

Asay, TP & Lambert, MJ (1999) Therapist relational variables. In DJ Cain & J Seeman (Eds) *Humanistic Psychotherapies: Handbook of theory and practice* (pp. 531–57). Washington, DC: American Psychological Association.

Attwood, T (2006) *The Complete Guide to Asperger's Syndrome*. London: Jessica Kingsley.

Baron, MG, Groden, J, Groden, G & Lipsitt, LP (Eds) (2006) *Stress and Coping in Autism*. Oxford: Oxford University Press.

Baron-Cohen, S (1995) *Mindblindness: An essay on autism and theory of mind*. Cambridge, MA: MIT Press.

Bauminger, N (2002) The facilitation of social-emotional understanding and social interaction in high-functioning children with autism: Intervention outcomes. *Journal of Autism and Developmental Disorders, 32*(4), 283–98.

Bauminger, N, Shulman, C & Agam, G (2003) Peer interaction and loneliness in high-functioning children with autism. *Journal of Autism and Developmental Disorders, 33*(5), 489–507.

Bowler, D (2007) *Autism Spectrum Disorders: Psychological theory and research*. Chichester: John Wiley & Sons.

Cardaciotto, L & Herbert, JD (2004) Cognitive behavior therapy for social anxiety disorder in the context of Asperger's syndrome: A single-subject report. *Cognitive and Behavioral Practice, 11*, 75–81.

Carrick, L & McKenzie, S (2011) A heuristic examination of the application of Pre-Therapy skills and the person-centered approach in the field of autism. *Person-Centered & Experiential Psychotherapies, 10*(2), 73–89.

Cooper, M (2008) *Essential Research Findings in Counselling and Psychotherapy: The facts are friendly*. London: Sage.

Cooper, M & McLeod, J (2007) A pluralistic framework for counselling and psychotherapy: Implications for research. *Counselling and Psychotherapy Research, 7*(3), 135–43.

Deudney, C & Shah, A (2001) *Mental Health and Asperger Syndrome – Information Sheet*. London: The National Autistic Society.

Ghaziuddin, M, Weidmer-Mihail, E & Ghaziuddin, N (1998) Comorbidity of Asperger syndrome: A preliminary report. *Journal of Intellectual Disability Research, 42*(4), 279–82.

Gillott, A, Furniss, F & Walter, A (2001) Anxiety in high-functioning children with autism. *Autism, 5*(3), 277–86.

Hamilton, AFdC, Brindley, RM & Frith, U (2007) Imitation and action understanding in autistic spectrum disorders: How valid is the hypothesis of a deficit in the mirror neuron system? *Neuropsychologia, 45*, 1859–68.

Hare, DJ, Jones, JPR & Paine, C (1999) Approaching reality: The use of personal construct assessment in working with people with Asperger syndrome. *Autism, 3*(2), 165–76.

Howlin, P (1997a) *Autism: Preparing for adulthood*. London: Routledge.

Howlin, P (1997b) Psychiatric disturbances in adulthood. In P Howlin (Ed) *Autism: Preparing for adulthood* (pp. 216–35). London: Routledge.

Jacob, P (2008) What do mirror neurons contribute to human social cognition? *Mind & Language, 23*(2), 190–223.

Kelly, AB, Garnett, MS, Attwood, T & Peterson, C (2008) Autism spectrum symptomatology in children: The impact of family and peer relationships. *J Abnorm Child Psychol, 36*, 1069–81.

Kim, JA, Szatmari, P, Bryson, SE, Streiner, DL & Wilson, FJ (2000) The prevalence of anxiety and mood problems among children with autism and Asperger syndrome. *Autism, 4*(2), 117–32.

King, M, Marston, L & Bower, P (2013) Comparison of non-directive counselling and cognitive behaviour therapy for patients presenting in general practice with an ICD-10 depressive episode: A randomized control trial. *Psychological Medicine*, Available on CJO 2013. doi: 10.1017/S0033291713002377

Knibbs, J, & Moran, H (2005) Autism and Asperger syndrome: Person-centred approaches. In S Joseph & R Worsley (Eds) *Person-Centred Psychopathology* (pp. 260–75). Ross-on-Wye: PCCS Books.

Luborsky, L, Diguer, L, Seligman, DA, Rosenthal, R, Krause, ED, Johnson, S et al (1999) The researcher's own therapy allegiances: A 'wild card' in comparisons of treatment efficacy. *Clinical Psychology: Science and Practice, 6*(1), 95–106.

Mero, M-M (2002) Asperger syndrome with comorbid emotional disorder – Treatment with psychoanalytic psychotherapy. *International Journal of Circumpolar Health, 61*(Suppl 2), 80–9.

Mitchell, P (1997) *Introduction to Theory of Mind: Children, autism and apes*. London: Arnold.

National Institute for Health and Care Excellence (2011) *Autism: Recognition, referral and diagnosis of children and young people on the autism spectrum*, CG128. London: NICE.

Norcross, JC (2002) *Psychotherapy Relationships that Work: Therapist contributions and responsiveness to patients*. Oxford: Oxford University Press.

Oliver, M (1990) *The Politics of Disablement*. Basingstoke: Macmillan.

Oliver, M (1996) *Understanding Disability: From theory to practice*. Basingstoke: Macmillan.

Petersilia, JR (2001) Crime victims with developmental disabilities: A review essay. *Criminal Justice and Behavior, 28*, 655–94.

Prouty, G, Van Werde, D & Pörtner, M (2002) *Pre-Therapy: Reaching contact-impaired clients*. Ross-on-Wye: PCCS Books.

Rogers, CR (1951) *Client-Centered Therapy: Its current practice, implications and theory*. London: Constable.

Sanders, P (Ed) (2012) *The Tribes of the Person-Centred Nation: An introduction to the schools of therapy related to the person-centred approach*. Ross-on-Wye: PCCS Books.

Sanders, P (2013) *Person-Centred Therapy Theory and Practice in the 21st Century*. Ross-on-Wye: PCCS Books.

Segrin, C (2001) *Interpersonal Processes in Psychological Problems*. New York: Guildford Press.

Schuurman, C (2010) *Cognitieve gedragstherapie bij autisme. Een praktisch behandelprogramma voor volwassenen*. Amsterdam: Hogrefe.

Sofronoff, K, Attwood, T & Hinton, S (2005) A randomised controlled trial of a CBT intervention for anxiety in children with Asperger syndrome. *Journal of Child Psychology and Psychiatry, 46*(11), 1152–60.

Sofronoff, K, Attwood, T, Hinton, S & Levin, I (2007) A randomized controlled trial of a cognitive behavioural intervention for anger management in children diagnosed with Asperger syndrome. *J Autism Dev Disord, 37*(7), 1203–14.

Spek, A (2010) *Mindfulness bij volwassenen met autisme. Een wegwijzer voor hulpverleners en mensen met ASS.* Amsterdam: Hogrefe.

Spek, AA, Ham, NC van & Lieshout, H van (2010) Effectiviteit van Mindfulness based stress reduction bij volwassenen met een autismespectrumstoornis. *Wetenschappelijk Tijdschrift Autisme, 9*(3), 82–8.

Stinckens, N & Becaus, L (2008) Opereren op vreemd grondgebied. Kennis als toegangspoort tot contact bij de stoornis van Asperger. *Tijdschrift Cliëntgerichte Psychotherapie, 46*(1), 17–37.

Tantam, D (2000) Psychological disorder in adolescents and adults with Asperger syndrome. *Autism, 4*(1), 47–62.

Vuijk, R (2013) Procesgerichte gesprekstherapie: enige gedachten over een procesbehandeling van normaal intelligente volwassenen met autismespectrumstoornissen (ASS). *Tijdschrift Cliëntgerichte Psychotherapie, 51*(2), 120–7.

Wampold, B (2001) *The Great Psychotherapy Debate: Models, methods and findings.* Mahwah, NJ: Erlbaum.

Warner, MS (2005) A person-centered view of human nature, wellness, and psychopathology. In S Joseph & R Worsley (Eds) *Person-Centred Psychopathology* (pp. 91–109). Ross-on-Wye: PCCS Books.

Warner, MS (2007) Client incongruence and psychopathology. In M Cooper, M O'Hara, P F Schmid & G Wyatt (Eds) *The Handbook of Person-Centred Psychotherapy and Counselling* (pp. 154–67). Basingstoke: Palgrave Macmillan.

White, SW & Roberson-Nay, R (2009) Anxiety, social deficits, and loneliness in youth with autism spectrum disorders. *J Autism Dev Disord, 39,* 1006–13.

Wing, L (1996) *The Autistic Spectrum.* London: Constable & Robinson.

8 Person-centred therapy for people with dementia

Danuta Lipinska

Living with dementia is viewed as one of the significant challenges of 21st-century life. We all know someone with dementia or someone who cares for a person with dementia. We are familiar with media campaigns and, increasingly, prominent personalities tell us their stories of living with dementia or caring for a loved one.

People with dementia are no longer willing to accept the designation of dementia victim or dementia sufferer, and neither should we, personally or professionally. Many people with dementia are writing and speaking at international conferences, or on radio and television, both about themselves, and about the challenges that come from living with the changes arising from dementia.

In such a life-altering situation, there are many men and women who would like to have the opportunity to engage in a professional counselling relationship in order to address their concerns and to attempt to make sense of self (Lipinska, 2009, p. 21).

Access to therapy for older people and especially those experiencing cognitive changes is a relatively recent development in the UK and an awareness of its importance and efficacy is only beginning to gain momentum.

This chapter is about person-centred therapy with people in the early and middle stages of dementia. The person-centred care for people with dementia in the later stages, when all aspects of the brain are severely affected, is described in the chapter by Penny Dodds et al., this volume.

Here I will briefly introduce the fundamentals of what dementia is and how a person may be affected. The person with dementia as client then becomes the focus and I describe possibilities and methods enabling person-centred therapy to flourish. In the face of an often ageist society, with consequent therapeutic and diagnostic nihilism for older people, it may seem something of an oxymoron to put the words 'dementia' and 'therapy' together in the same sentence. The belief that therapy takes place with significant outcomes for clients with dementia may fly in the face of accepted therapeutic wisdom, and challenge what we thought we knew about the relationship between neurobiology and the ability to create meaningful therapeutic relationships in spite of, or because of, multiple changes in a person's life and experience of self.

What is dementia?

Dementia is the name given to a collection or cluster of symptoms or behaviours and experiences which indicate that brain cells are dying prematurely. All aspects of being, functioning and relating; from the simplest to most complex tasks are eventually going to be affected. In the present state of research, we cannot prevent or cure the conditions which give rise to the three most common forms of dementia: Alzheimer's disease, dementia with Lewy bodies (DLB) and vascular dementia.

Even in times of extreme distress, I take for granted the smooth running of a functional brain, in particular, functioning memory, to allow me to make sense of the world and my abilities, communication, my past, present and future, and how to look after my self within its current context.

There exists a pervasive myth that all experiences of dementia are negative and based on disintegration, degeneration, diminishment and despair; that any form of dementia renders the individual at once completely incapable, dysfunctional, non-communicative and unreachable. The person with dementia is imagined from the outset as the dependent resident in a care home. Although this is sometimes eventually the case, it is not always so, especially in the early stages, and men and women live and die at home and in their own communities. Our tendency to stereotype and our quest to assess and measure the effects of dementia on the brain and behaviour and the therapeutic process can lead us in a direction of misinformation and 'malignant social psychology' as Tom Kitwood describes our negative attitudes, responses and lowered expectations of people with dementia within our society (Kitwood, 1997, p. 4).

A daughter describes her experience in this way:

> When my mother was given a mental status test several months before entering a nursing home, her score was zero. Her family knew that she still had cognition, but not the kind addressed on the test. Examples of the questions were: How old are you? Where is this place located? Who is the President of the United States? These were precisely representative of the things she no longer knew. What did she know? Things I could not put into words at the time. She understood textures, fabrics, sunsets, birds at the bird feeder, friendly faces – when something was wrong. She knew me. She just didn't remember my name. (Whitcomb, 1986)

In a world more demanding of the rigours of science to provide evidence for what the impaired brain can no longer achieve, and how we might pursue a cure, the medical community is often confounded by the strengths that remain in the lives of men and women with dementia. The subtleties of nuance and metaphor in communication, newly developed creativity and an appreciation for the spiritual and life in the 'here and now' cannot be underestimated or overlooked. So too, in the therapeutic realm, the demand for assessment, measurement, and evidence of the benefits of therapy leave little room for the powerful self-reporting from clients, their partners, families and the professionals who support them as they share the unexpected impact of therapy in the life of the person with dementia.

In his searching and stimulating book, *The Soul of Counseling*, Dwight Webb writes:

> The *soul* cannot be captured by boundary markers. No net may be cast to contain it. In therapeutic counseling there is no linear or quantitative measurement of the soul. We need to acknowledge that we don't have to measure everything. An act of kindness, for example, is a spiritual gift, and is to be experienced with savouring and rejoicing. Why try to reduce it to numbers? Such natural acts of love are too full of wonder to quantify. (Webb, 2005, p. 99)

> In the UK over 750,000 men and women over the age of 65 have dementia and approximately 17,000 under the age of 65 have more rare forms of dementia. (Alzheimer Society Fact Sheets)

Dementia is not a normal part of ageing, and those of us who are not yet considered 'old' are not exempt from its arrival. The dementias of early onset are not the most common occurrences of dementia in the population, but increased diagnosis has emphatically highlighted the issue that these conditions are not necessarily about 'getting old and losing your mind' but more about a range of neurological conditions affecting adults, where old age is but one of the risk factors.

My youngest client has been a woman of 38, a married school teacher with two young children. Demographics in the Western world show a steadily ageing population, and as dementia classically affects men and women over 65 (1 in 10) with a steep rise from age 80 (1 in 5) onwards more people will be affected in our lifetimes and dementia will increasingly become part of our most intimate partnerships, families, friendships and communities. The challenges of supporting individuals and families have changed too and often there are four-generational households. The primary carer of the person with dementia may be, for example, either 85 years old and caring for an adult child with HIV-AIDS-related dementia or 13 years of age, caring for a grandparent whose adult son or daughter (the father or mother) is dead, absent, unwell or struggling with addiction or mental health concerns.

This also means that as therapists we must be aware of and prepare for the 21st-century client, and increasingly those from the so-called 'baby boomer' generation who will have had a very different experience of therapy and counselling than the previous two generations.

Although confusion, memory loss and difficulties with language and everyday activities like bathing, dressing, cooking and driving gradually become more challenging, we know that people with dementia can manage to function in spite of these changes with the support of others. Kitwood describes how, paradoxically, verbal and non-verbal communication may, for a time, become clearer and more direct as the person's inhibition of social engagement becomes less.

> People who have dementia and for whom the life of the emotions is often intense, and without the ordinary forms of inhibition, may have something important to teach the rest of humankind. (Kitwood, 1997, p. 34)

For a time, the vulnerable individual may emerge from behind their 'mask' as someone fiercely alive, authentic and real and perhaps capable of quite staggering interactions, relationships and experiences, if only the time can be taken to be there to listen and encourage them with heart and spirit. This is never easy for a partner or family member with whom the person has a history, an intense emotional and spiritual connection and a radically altered future.

I have found it humbling and incredible to witness the myriad ways in which persons with dementia forge a path through confusion, chaos and memory loss. In many instances, creative abilities in particular develop in the most magnificent and surprising ways not consistent with what we would expect from a supposedly degenerative condition. Much has been captured in the literature as creative arts such as photography, painting, dance, art, poetry, film and music.

Renowned British author, Terry Pratchett, when he was 59 and diagnosed with a rare form of Alzheimer's disease, posterior cortical atrophy (PCA), said:

> Frankly, I would prefer it if people kept things cheerful, because I think there's time for at least a few more books yet. I will, of course, be dead at some future point, as will everybody else. For me, this may be further off than you think – it's too soon to tell. (Pratchett, 2007)

Indeed, two books have been published since he made this statement.

Nick's Misericords, a film made by Nick Jones, describes his experience of dementia and a new-found love and talent for drawing. Perhaps much of this focuses on what we would call right-hemisphere functioning. Although all aspects of the brain will ultimately be affected, those creative, emotional and spiritual areas of ability, expression and engagement, mainly specialised in the right hemisphere which may previously have been under-developed, can come to the fore, can be encouraged and celebrated.

Who is the client?

The person with dementia is a unique individual with a past present and a future. He or she will also have a unique experience and expression of their form of dementia. As Christine Boden (1997, pp. 49–50) states: 'The unique essence of "me" is at my core, and this is what will remain with me at the end. I will perhaps be more truly "me" than I have ever been.'

In my nearly 30 years of experience, both in the UK and the USA, I have been struck that irrespective of the age of the client, their type of dementia, or where they are in their experience of it, there seems to be an ardent, if not urgent desire to 'make sense of self' – the self in its interiority; what goes on within and is often hidden; its exteriority; what goes on in the external world; and its relativity, the relationship between both, mediated by the emotional and spiritual.

The reasons that bring any client to the intimacies of a therapeutic relationship with a professionally trained stranger are the same for the person with dementia. Time and again, I have witnessed the additional concerns that somehow partners, relatives or friends will not know how to handle what the client might need to share. This includes their fears and anxieties for the future or of the multiple changes, losses and grief consistent with a more dependent lifestyle, an unwelcome future and eventual death.

I have found the description below particularly helpful. It can be applied equally to persons with dementia as to any other clients:

> In the here and now exploration, clients also have an opportunity to find out from a (congruent) other how they are experienced, and this can help them develop their ability to engage with others as they actually are, rather than as the client might imagine them to be. (Mearns & Cooper, 2005, p. 134)

Often people will ask how I expect therapy to be helpful, when the client might not remember my name, may miss the session, may forget where they parked the car or what was said last week. I agree that these aspects of forgetfulness could be problematic, but not any more than my experience of some clients who do not have dementia. We have more in common than we imagine, and therefore can enter into the therapeutic relationship with the same care and anticipation as ever we would.

One client told me: 'I need to tell you my story – before I forget the words.' Indeed, the use of narrative can be an extremely potent and poignant part of the client's self-expression. Oliver Sacks, the neurologist, famous for striving to reach the unreachable, says:

> We have, each of us, a life-story, an inner narrative – whose continuity, whose sense, is our lives. It might be said that each one of us constructs and lives a 'narrative' and that this narrative is us, our identities. To be ourselves, we must have ourselves – possess, if need be, re-possess our life-stories. We must 'recollect' ourselves; recollect the inner drama, the narrative, of ourselves. A man needs such a narrative, a continuous inner narrative, to maintain his identity, his self. (Sacks, 1988, p. 34)

As I have listened to my clients' narratives on numerous occasions, it has seemed of vital importance to the client to re-member and re-assemble their functional self, and for us both to acknowledge not only what has been, but what is and what is still to come.

The person-centred approach

Over many years of therapeutic work with clients with dementia I have begun to develop language to describe the theoretical framework upon which we have been building our particular therapeutic 'domain'.

Invariably, clients describe living with dementia in terms of their emotional, psychological and spiritual experience and I am invited to be 'within the experiencing' (Mearns & Thorne, 2000), not outside of it. Unbeknown to me, the client may be presenting his or her perception of self rather than the self than actually loses the car keys, puts his clothes on inside out or forgets how to get home from the shopping centre. These various authentic selves are not dissociated states, but rather the many and sometimes conflicting/contradictory experiences of a person with variations in cognitive functioning and emotional being. Relatives have often pointed out that I do not see or hear the person with whom they live and see deteriorating before their eyes. Although that may well be true, the therapeutic relationship has always been a place for exploring parts of the self, some of which are known only to the self and perhaps now to the therapist also.

The importance of confidentiality is paramount. Often relatives and health and social care workers believe that we are all in the same circle of confidentiality and have the best interests of the client/patient at heart. I believe the quality of my commitment to confidentiality enables the client to more freely enter into the relationship, safe in the knowledge that I will not share what they tell me (apart from under the usual conditions). It encourages honesty, integrity and the possibility of relational depth.

The collaborative writing of Mearns and Thorne (2000) for me validated the process that had been taking place in countless relationships, in two countries; often in direct contradiction to the usual expectations for people living with mild to moderate cognitive change and loss. My initial surprise has been sustained as I observe that change and growth are possible and even highly likely if Rogers' core conditions of empathy, unconditional positive regard and congruence can be offered regardless of cognitive limitations.

In addition to the core conditions, taking the risk to work at 'relational depth', with 'configurations of self' and in 'not-for-growth areas' (Mearns & Thorne, 2000), encourages us both to stay focused and welcoming of whatever the client brings. Staying present to the client in this pull towards a worsening condition, loss of control and choice and ultimately, death, can give rise to experiences we do not usually expect. Clients have described feeling truly heard and affirmed, and discovering feelings of wellbeing, confidence, security, value and the ability to make themselves known and heard by others.

> Indeed some of the most absorbing person-centred work occurs when the client is at the pre-symbolic stage in relation to a configuration of self. Here, the client and therapist cannot talk about the configuration; they can only be in the configuration. The client is dimly and partially expressing himself from the configuration but the material is not neatly organized. For the therapist whose listening requires coherence there is only confusion. What is required is a listening that hears the person rather than the content. The listening is to the existence and expressing of the person. It is the expressing which is being listened to rather than the expression. (Mearns & Thorne, 2000, p. 129)

Here are a few statements from men and women who have been clients:

> You have really helped me to get control of myself and what's happening to me.

> When I talk to you, I feel a whole weight lifting off me.

> I never thought I could ever forgive him, but talking to you about it has really helped me to do it!

Clients are able to forgive and experience resolution if given the opportunity and the desire to do so.

> I could never tell my wife how I feel; she has so much to deal with just looking out for me.

> It's not just the talking, it's the silence too.

> I know I can talk to my family, but counselling gives me the chance to have some time for myself to talk openly about what is bothering me that I wouldn't want to share with them. I'm still my own person and I don't want them to know all my secrets.

> She is much more relaxed when she has been to see you and seems to sleep better at night.

> You will never know how much the sessions have meant to him and to me. I just couldn't cope with all he had to get off his chest.

> It has given her peace of mind again. She doesn't tell me what you talk about and I don't ask. We just both know it's better.

More detailed accounts and reflections of the statements of not only clients, but their relatives and the professionals who support them, can be found elsewhere (Lipinska, 2009).

How does therapy work?

If we appreciate that talking therapies are known to reduce feelings of depression, isolation and anxiety and that neural pathways can be strengthened and new ones created, there is hope that therapy can offer the very same thing for people with dementia.

From the outset clients need to come to therapy voluntarily. In this work I may need to re-introduce myself, what we are doing together, what time we meet and ensure that the client does want to stay and talk with me. One client said that I was 'the keeper of the memories'. It makes sense that I would be the one to offer those conversations and themes anew as a way of re-establishing contact.

This can also save the client the time and embarrassment of searching for the unremembered. Clients will receive the same information regarding the therapeutic contract and confidentiality along with a discussion about and how they wish me to interact with their partner or relative and arrange appointments if the partner or relative is bringing them to sessions. We will discuss what therapy is, who I am, the training I have received, my supervision and what our relationship might be like.

As in all situations, according to the Mental Capacity Act (2005), we are to assume that a person has the capacity to make decisions regarding their life and relationships unless indicated otherwise by formal assessment. I will re-establish the conditions of working, for example, my name and my role, if the client wishes to meet, when and where we shall meet, for how long and the role of confidentiality at the beginning and end of each session, always giving the client the opportunity to end at any time, even within the session.

As dementias are progressive and degenerative conditions, the person's abilities and desire to remain in the room or in the relationship may change over time and I will review with them how sessions are going for them at each new session, being especially observant of changes in communication or attention or any signs of distress, anxiety or discomfort.

In some circumstances the client will move to live with a relative, into a care home or sadly, may die before we have ended therapy. It is therefore particularly important that the therapist has ongoing professional supervision, reflective practice and self-care strategies if this kind of work is to be undertaken.

The pace and content of the session will be established by the client and I strive to stay alert to the subtleties of non-verbal behaviour especially facial expressions, body movement and posture, sometimes mirroring the client, expressing what I sense in my body and reflecting this back to them. Here is an example with Bill:

> Danuta: I'm looking at your face and at your eyes. You seem so sad.
>
> Bill: [nods]
>
> D: Your body is kind of slumped, like this [mirroring his position and facial

expression]. It looks like a heavy burden and feels like one to me too.

[Silence as we sit, mirror images of one another.]

B: Stupid, feels stupid. I'm stupid.

D: You're feeling stupid and that's kind of embarrassing? When your boss would get mad at you in front of your friends? [He's nodding, but not moving.] Like maybe how it is when your memory doesn't work like you want it to?

B: Yeah. [BIG sigh]

D: That's a big sigh Bill, from way down deep [I sigh like he did]. It feels like here ... [I put my fist in my gut].

B: [Looks right at me and straightens a little.] That's right.

D: [Nodding slowly.] Right.

[Silence]

D: I think I get what you want to say Bill. Can I try and say it back to you?

B: Yeah, OK.

D: OK. Stop me if I get it wrong or go too fast. The feeling you get when your memory doesn't work is like how you felt around your boss when he was mad at you?

B: Nodding.

D: You feel stupid, embarrassed?

B: Yep. [Moving now, changing position but still making himself small in the chair.]

D: Is it like shame?

B: [Looking down and away.] Yes, that's it. Shame. I feel ashamed.

D: [Nodding.] Mmmm ...

B: Stupid and ashamed. I can't do anything about it.

(Lipinska, 2009, pp. 98–9)

We were able to continue to explore the themes of his feeling anxious and stupid and how he might like to regain some control over situations like this one. When I asked what he would like to say to his boss, or to other people, Bill was able to say that he would tell people up front: 'Hey, my memory doesn't work the way it used to [and then chuckling, with a boyish grin on his face, added], so take it easy on me, OK?' This seemingly simple strategy empowered Bill to have control over his memory lapses and word-finding difficulties which left him tongue-tied, embarrassed and wanting to withdraw emotionally and leave the room.

We can see here the ability to engage with humour and wit which can remain intact for a long time. Humour can often be a way in which people with dementia can engage more playfully and light-heartedly with their feelings and experiences. This often gives others permission to do the same. Working in a group of men with dementia some years ago, the men decided that when they were stuck for words they would say they had 'brain cramp' and they laughed long and hard and used the term frequently.

Humour and laughter also release much-needed endorphins or 'feel good' chemicals in the brain, which have positive felt and observed results.

This exchange with Janet, a retired law professor with Parkinson's disease, is an example of how we co-created our communication and how the time she had to herself in the session allowed her to reach her anger and speak the unspeakable in my presence:

> Danuta: I can see how much effort this is for you, Janet. I really want to be able to hear your concerns and to support you the best way I can. Would it be OK if we talk a bit about how we can communicate the best way for you and for us both?
>
> Janet: It takes too long. [These few words took several seconds accompanied by much contortion of facial muscles, drooling and her wiping her mouth in between.]
>
> D: [Nods.] For you or for others?
>
> J: Mainly me. No one waits long enough to hear.
>
> D: No one waits long enough to hear you?
>
> J: [Nods, looking sad.]
>
> D: It seems to make you sad, not being heard, not being given time.
>
> J: [Nods, still looking sad.]
>
> D: I would really like to hear you. [Pause.] I have time to hear you now. [Pause.] We can meet for an hour every week if you would like and we can take our time.
>
> J: [Nodding and smiling slightly.] I'd really like that. [Again this took several seconds with much the same process as before, with great effort and wiping her mouth.]
>
> D: You'd like that? And I would too. [Pause.] How would it be if I help you with a word if you seem stuck, or if I go over something to make sure I understand you? You can tell me to stop or to 'shut up' any time if you find it annoying. How does that sound to you?
>
> J: [Smiling, head tilted to one side, eyebrows raised.] We could try it.
>
> D: OK, we'll try it. What would you like to talk about today Janet?
>
> J: My daughter. I'm so angry at her. She thinks I'm HER daughter! [Voice is raised and she looks angry too, this has taken her about 30 seconds as she also dropped her hankie down the side of the chair and had to get it back out again.] Tell her to go back to Chicago. She's driving me CRAZY!
>
> D: You're angry with your daughter? [Pause.] She's driving you crazy? [Pause.] How is that?
>
> J: [Nods.] She tells me what to do all the time. Treats me like an idiot.
>
> D: It sounds as if she's being the one in charge and treats you like you don't know anything?
>
> J: That's right. [Nodding slowly.]
>
> (Lipinska, 2009, pp. 93–4)

Janet had been heard and acknowledged without being judged. More importantly, time was essential for her to gather her thoughts and allow the physical demands needed to sit relatively still and form the words and movements required to get her tongue and mouth to cooperate.

Janet eventually invited her daughter to a session where she was able to tell her some of her concerns and feelings: that she would prefer her daughter to go back to Chicago and that Janet would have more support at home. Mother and daughter established a routine of regular long-weekend visits at Janet's home and they had various enjoyable outings and friends over for coffee or a meal.

In such a situation it may be all too easy for the therapist to find themselves talking to Janet's daughter on her behalf. Other health and social care professionals might consider it wise to intervene in order to preserve the relationship between the two. The outcome as we see it here empowered Janet and her residual strengths and abilities and helped her daughter to see her mother as still independent and capable in spite of obvious changes and needs. It allowed them to co-create a new dimension to their relationship.

In some cases, a client has been able to state that counselling is not helpful. A lady, resident in a care home, expressed that after the session ended she was left alone with a whole range of emotions and nothing to do but feel awful. She was able to say that she would rather not delve into the sadness of her lost relationship with her son and requested that someone should please fix her up with lots of things to do to take her mind off it completely. With her permission a visit from a social worker and an activities coordinator was arranged and an individualised schedule was prepared according to her needs and interests.

Clients are sometimes seen at their residential care home, day centre or occasionally in their own home. Clients drive themselves to therapy in their own cars, cycle, arrange for taxis or lifts from family or friends, and use public transportation. Much of my work has been part of my long-standing private practice, and clients are often in charge of their own finances or tell me who is going to be paying my fee if it is not them.

Spiritual aspects of the relationship

More often than I would have imagined, therapeutic relationships with men and women living with dementia in various stages and differing forms has taken place on several levels. The most intriguing has been the engagement at the spiritual level. In some cases this has been part of the person's lifelong religious practice, in others, a sublime and highly evocative transcendent experience between us.

My experience brings to mind Carl Rogers' words:

> A vast and mysterious universe – perhaps an inner reality, or perhaps a
> spirit world of which we are all unknowingly a part – seems to exist. Such a

> universe delivers a final crushing blow to our comfortable belief that we all
> know what the real world is. (Rogers, 1978, p. 8)

Spirituality can be a sustaining, affirming and comforting aspect of the self which allows for control and hope to be placed in the hands if a divine 'other' for safekeeping. Each of us as therapists must assess how much we can allow ourselves to be open to our own spirituality and how this may respond to or invite the spiritual in our client. This exchange could take the form of the client describing life events with particular spiritual nuance: nature, poetry, the birth of a child, a favourite piece of music or art, a relationship with a lover, child or friend.

There are many recorded examples of men and women across various faith traditions, some with severe limitations to spoken communication, who have been able to sing many verses of hymns and chants, recite sacred texts and take part in rituals with apparent engagement, enjoyment and meaning. We know that the memory for singing and music is surprisingly often available, but the additional spiritual dimension with its combination of emotional and sensory material may help to embed these particular types of memories and their expression. The close relationship between creativity and spirituality has been explored by many including myself (2009), Goldsmith (1996), Killick (2006), MacKinlay (2008), Jewell (2011), and MacKinlay and Trevitt (2012).

Brian Thorne illuminates this notion expertly:

> My spirit and your spirit are what ultimately define us; it is our spirit that gives meaning and direction to our experience. It is our spirit that determines our identity and it is our spirit which bears the mark of immortality. We are body, mind and spirit, but it is the spirit that breathes life and gives light – or colludes with death and darkness. The existentialists' question 'who am I?' can only be satisfactorily answered in terms of the spirit. (Thorne, 1998, p. 151)

For persons with dementia, the questions may become less philosophical and more pertinent to their actual existence. To answer the question 'who am I?' with the obvious in terms of person, place and time becomes not only unhelpful but borders on the patronising.

The person at times may truly believe themselves to be the 11-year-old at school and of course they would not then be Mrs Brown and would not have a husband or five children as we know to be the case. Many years ago, 'reality orientation' was the order of the day until we finally discovered that it made little difference to the person what day of the week it was, but it left them and the professionals in a state of heightened anxiety and negativity, as many of the answers to the supposedly orientating were consistently incorrect. Without colluding with hallucinations or delusions, we have learned from Naomi Feil's 'Validation Therapy' (Feil, 1982) that communication can be enhanced through sensitive and patient observation, saying aloud what we hear and see, and reflecting back the feelings beneath the words and the behaviour. This approach affirms the individual and their experiencing rather than my imposing my idea of what reality should be. The emotional/spiritual content of the person's experience then provides a relevant bridge to communication which may lead to the heart of the distress or joy.

In conclusion

What seems for me to emerge through the various narratives and relationships is the pervasive presence and essence of love. It is perhaps no coincidence that in the last years of his life, Rogers wrote more about the therapist-offered condition of unconditional positive regard as love. The late Tom Kitwood, founder of person-centred care of people with dementia, places love unapologetically at the centre of his requirements for psychological wellbeing in persons with dementia. It is essential that we allow the person with dementia as client to give as well as receive, and in more situations than I imagined possible, at the end of the agreed therapy, clients have told me that they love me, and in all honesty I have been able to tell them the same.

We are daily being challenged to acknowledge our own fears, stereotypes and misgivings about our approach to people with dementia, our views of dementia, and the needs and wants of the individuals whose lives it affects. Let us also be willing to acknowledge the fruits of our continued joint endeavours for more open communication, exploration and research, as we work towards the development of appropriate alternative support and therapies, outside the realms of the disease model, which normalises and de-pathologises dementia.

It is my hope and my privilege to continue to share my experiences in therapeutic relationships with people with dementia over a 30-year period, both in the USA and the UK and to offer encouragement and a foundation for newly emerging therapists or those already in practice to include men and women experiencing the life-altering conditions associated with cognitive change.

I firmly believe that faced with the complexities of living with dementia and, ultimately, the challenges of its effects on verbal communication, people with dementia who would like to have professional counselling need it to be available within their local community.

The 'difficult edge' for me is not that therapy with persons with dementia is not possible or valuable, but that it is yet in its infancy. I look forward with excited anticipation as therapeutic relationships with men and women with dementia come of age in the not too distant future.

References

Alzheimer's Society Fact Sheets 400–4. Retrieved 25 February 2014 from www.alzheimers.org. uk/factsheets

Boden, C (1997) *Who Will I Be When I Die?* London: HarperCollins.

Feil, N (1982) *V/F Validation: The Feil Method.* Cleveland, OH: Edward Feil Press.

Goldsmith, M (1996) *Hearing the Voice of People with Dementia: Opportunities and obstacles.* London & Philadelphia: Jessica Kingsley Publishers.

Jewell, A (2011) *Spirituality and Personhood in Dementia.* London & Philadelphia: Jessica Kingsley Publishers.

Jones, N (2010) *Nick's Misericords.* Innovations in Dementia. Retrieved 25 February 2014 from www.innovationsindementia.org.uk

Killick, J (2006) Helping the flame to stay bright: Celebrating the spiritual in dementia. *Journal of Religion, Spirituality and Ageing, 18*(2/3), 73.

Kitwood, T (1997) *Dementia Reconsidered: The person comes first.* Buckingham: Open University Press.

Lipinska, D (2009) *Person-Centred Counselling for People with Dementia: Making sense of self.* London & Philadelphia: Jessica Kingsley Publishers.

MacKinlay, E (2008) *Ageing and Spirituality across Faiths and Cultures.* London & Philadelphia: Jessica Kingsley Publishers.

MacKinlay, E & Trevitt, C (2012) *Finding Meaning in the Experience of Dementia: The place of spiritual reminiscence work.* London & Philadelphia: Jessica Kingsley Publishers.

Mearns, D & Cooper, M (2005) *Working at Relational Depth in Counselling and Psychotherapy.* London: Sage Publications.

Mearns, D & Thorne, B (2000) *Person-Centred Therapy Today: New frontiers in theory and practice.* London: Sage Publications.

Mental Capacity Act (2005) Retrieved 22nd April 2014 from http://www.legislation.gov.uk/ukpga/2005/9/contents

Pratchett, T (2007) Terry Pratchett: I Have Alzheimer's. *The Times Online,* retrieved 22nd April 2014 from http://boingboing.net/2007/12/12/terry-pratchett-has.html

Rogers, CR (1978) Do we need a reality? *Dawnpoint, 1*(2), 6–9.

Sacks, O (1988) *The Man Who Mistook His Wife for a Hat.* New York: Harper & Row.

Thorne, B (1998) *Person-Centred Counselling and Christian Spirituality: The secular and the holy.* London: Whurr Publishers.

Webb, D (2005) *The Soul of Counseling.* Atascadero, CA: Impact Publishers.

Whitcomb, J (1986) Is the glass half empty or half full? *American Journal of Alzheimer's Care and Related Disorders, 1*(2), 9–14.

Pre-Therapy and dementia – the opportunity to put Person-Centred theory into everyday practice

9

Penny Dodds, Pamela Bruce-Hay and Sally Stapleton

> I can't ... it all just falls off from me ...and wherever it is ... oh I just don't know anymore. (conversation with a man who was not able to introduce himself as he was unable to recall his name)

This chapter will locate Garry Prouty's Pre-Therapy amongst approaches in dementia care which are both broadly 'person-focused' and Person-Centred. Specifically, it will show the use of Prouty's Pre-Therapy contact work which, with origins in Person-Centred Therapy (Rogers, 1959; Sanders, 2007), has offered an additional approach to working with people with dementia for those striving to practise in a Person-Centred way (Prouty et al., 2002; Prouty, 2008).

The focus is on people with moderate or significant levels of dementia. They face challenges from cognitive changes, which in turn pose challenges to staff wishing to communicate and offer care. People with advanced levels of dementia have difficulties with maintaining the same understanding of the world around them as those who do not have dementia. Frequently, people with dementia are disoriented in time, reliving and talking about past experiences and memories as if in the present, sometimes with great temporal fluidity. Non-verbal and emotional communication increases in significance in later dementia with less focus on the exact content of communication, and more focus on meaning and emotional tones of conversations. Language is frequently disturbed, correct words may be difficult to find, syntax and grammar may be affected and sentences become disjointed. Patterns of speech may become more metaphorical and abstract, making it difficult for workers to grasp meanings and understand the world of the person with dementia as they are experiencing it. To inhabit this world must be a perplexing and at times, frustrating experience, particularly when those around do not seem to understand and cannot seem to communicate effectively.

We would like to thank Emma Day, trainee clinical psychologist, for sharing her work and providing a transcript.

Hey you, with that one, can you help as mmmmm there's two factions down there and I've not had any of it ... will it, with it? Come on Harry.

However, the challenges of working therapeutically with people who have a significant level of cognitive impairment are not insurmountable. A range of approaches and techniques exist, which indicate that meaningful contact and relationships are possible.

The landscape of Person-Centred therapeutic approaches and person-centred care

For the purpose of this chapter we need clarity around the terms 'person-centred care' and 'person-centred approaches' and locate these in relation to Person-Centred Therapy or therapeutic approaches grounded in the Person-Centred tradition. For simplicity, we use 'person-centred' (lower case) for the broad and general meaning of being attentive to an individual and 'Person-Centred' (upper case) for the more specific approaches which are Rogerian in origin and more closely tied to the Person-Centred Therapy tradition. Pre-Therapy is identified as a bridge between them. This is explained below and summarised in Figure 1 on p. 104.

There is terminological confusion around the term 'person-centred' in the dementia arena in the UK. Used as a broad term, it underpins the aspirations of an organisational culture to ensure the individual is at the heart of care, or provides a conceptual framework which embraces a philosophy of the humanity of caring (McCormack et al., 2011; McCance et al., 2011). The term also encompasses a wide range of 'person-centred care' practices. These hold the intention of being generally therapeutic and oriented towards placing the person at the centre of care as opposed to care which is task oriented or not focused on individual's needs – for example, encouraging activities, reminiscence, engagement using movement or music, use of dolls, touch and massage. Within 'person-centred care' the intention is to offer life-enhancing ways of being and interacting which enhance or engage with the lived experience of the person with dementia.

Many of the person-centred care approaches in dementia care deviate from what would be identified as Person-Centred from a Rogerian perspective in theory or practice, for example, Validation Therapy (Feil & De Klerk-Rubin, 2012). In Validation Therapy, the client's experience of reality is not questioned or corrected, rather the worker strives to enter into their world and jointly explore the world further. Whilst the relational aspects draw heavily on Rogerian principles, the underlying theoretical perspective is psychoanalytic, drawing on Erik Erikson's psychosocial developmental stages, itself a development of Freudian thinking. In Validation Therapy, the navigation of life stages, resolution of past events, and the final task of managing the conflict between maintaining ego

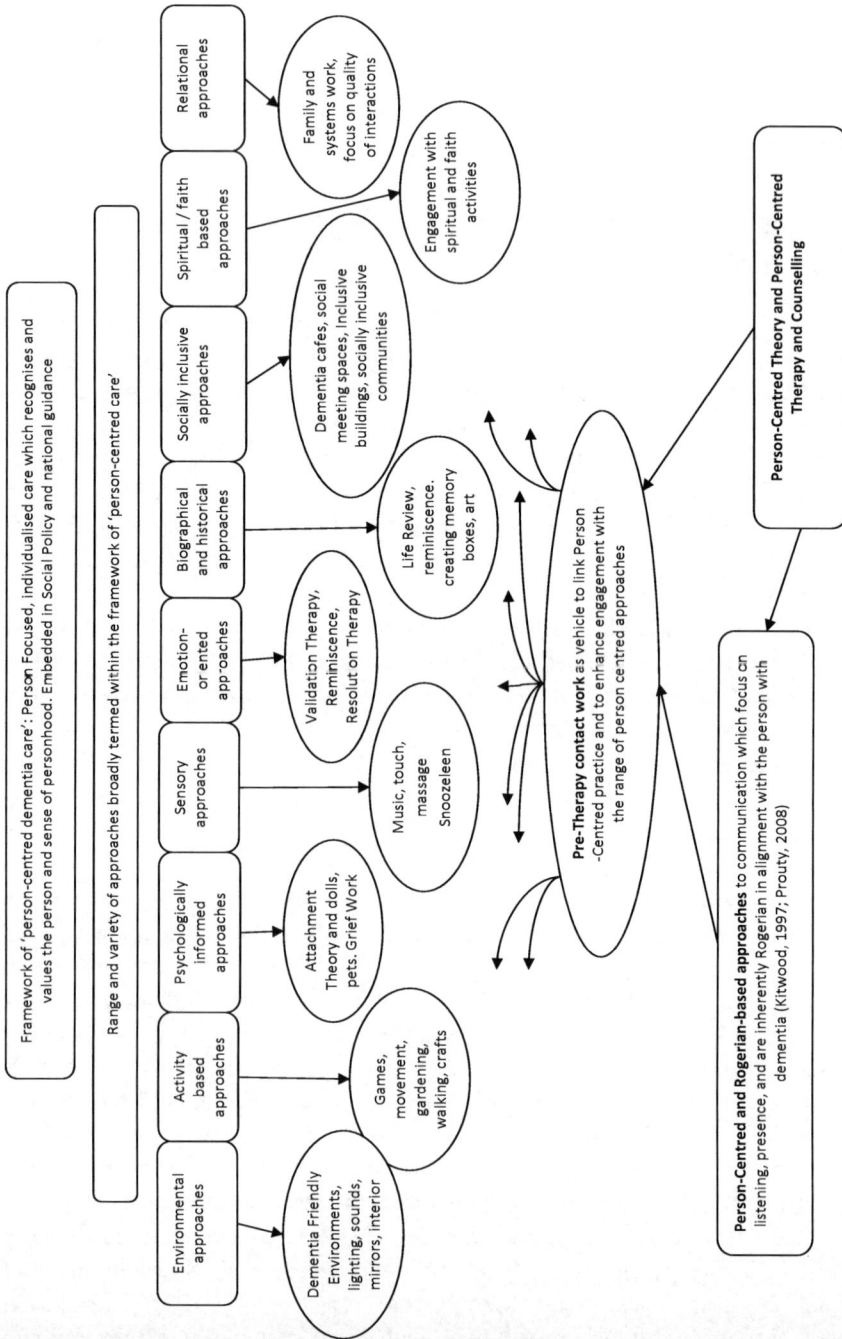

Figure 1. The landscape of Person-Centred and person-centred approaches in dementia care

Framework of 'person-centred dementia care': Person Focused, individualised care which recognises and values the person and sense of personhood. Embedded in Social Policy and national guidance

Range and variety of approaches broadly termed within the framework of 'person-centred care'

Environmental approaches

Dementia Friendly Environments, lighting, sounds, mirrors, interior

Activity based approaches

Games, movement, gardening, walking, crafts

Psychologically informed approaches

Attachment Theory and dolls, pets. Grief Work

Sensory approaches

Music, touch, massage Snoozeleen

Emotion-oriented approaches

Validation Therapy, Reminiscence, Resolut on Therapy

Biographical and historical approaches

Life Review, reminiscence. creating memory boxes, art

Socially inclusive approaches

Dementia cafes, social meeting spaces, inclusive buildings, socially inclusive communities

Spiritual / faith based approaches

Engagement with spiritual and faith activities

Relational approaches

Family and systems work, focus on quality of interactions

Pre-Therapy contact work as vehicle to link Person-Centred practice and to enhance engagement with the range of person centred approaches

Person-Centred Theory and Person-Centred Therapy and Counselling

Person-Centred and Rogerian-based approaches to communication which focus on listening, presence, and are inherently Rogerian in alignment with the person with dementia (Kitwood, 1997; Prouty, 2008)

integrity against despair form part of the theoretical background to interactions which help explore the meaning of the world for the person with dementia.

Amongst the mosaic of ways of providing 'person-centred care', some are more akin to a Person-Centred therapeutic approach. Like an umbilical cord, these approaches form the link between Rogerian theoretical origins and the more generalised 'person-centred' dementia care movement. A number of authors offer a recognisably Person-Centred approach with humanist origins. Tom Kitwood and Kathleen Bredin explicitly reference Rogers:

> We called the whole approach 'person-centred care', following the example of Rogerian psychotherapy. (Kitwood, 1997, p. 4)

Kitwood outlined interactions used to support an individual's personhood, which he termed *Positive Person Work*. These have been expanded by Brooker and Surr (2005) to include a list of 17 *personal enhancers*. Within this list are warmth, respect, acceptance and genuineness, which have clear links to Rogers' core conditions. Attending to the person and offering a presence allied with the humanist tradition is also evident in the emphasis on the relational demands of working with people with dementia (Greenwood, 2007) and in the work of Cheston (1998) whose psychotherapeutic work is explicit about attending, empathic listening and *bearing witness* to the person with dementia.

Another addition to Person-Centred practice which has been used in dementia care is Garry Prouty's Pre-Therapy (Prouty et al., 2002; Sanders, 2007; Van Werde & Prouty, 2013). This adds to the repertoire of practice which bridges 'person-centred care' and Person-Centred practice.

Pre-Therapy with people with dementia

Van Werde and Morton introduced Pre-Therapy to the field of dementia in the UK, identifying it as having potential as emotional palliative care (Van Werde & Morton, 1999). Pre-Therapy takes the starting point that, due to psychological distress or disturbance, people may be *out of contact*, meaning that they are less able or unable to engage with others as they struggle with, or lose contact with, their sense of self or experienced self; they have *lost touch* with the reality around them such as their situation or environment; and their capacity to communicate with others in the world is compromised. Together these create a state of *loss of contact* or a state of being *pre-expressive*.

Prouty's work focuses on the need for a client to have, or re-establish, contact, or have sufficient strength of contact before therapy can occur – hence the term *Pre-Therapy*. It is this focus on the establishment of contact which leads to the specific and concrete techniques used to restore contact and help people become more in touch with themselves, their situation and their capacity for communication. When used in more general care settings, not specifically preparing people for psychotherapy, Prouty calls this 'contact work' (Sanders, 2007).

Prouty's Pre-Therapy has clear theoretical, philosophical and conceptual foundations (Prouty et al., 2002), including Person-Centred psychology origins (Rogers, 1951), experiential focus (Gendlin, 1973), existential phenomenology and Merleau-Ponty's concept of embodiment (Merleau-Ponty, 2002). Whilst the foundations are important, it is the practical application and the use of contact work that appeals to us and is the subject of this chapter.

Contact work holds the potential for staff in dementia care to enact person-centredness in their everyday work. Staff caring for people with moderate and severe dementia, whether in residential homes or supported in the community, generally have little or no training and experience of psychotherapy or counselling practice. The reflections which form contact work provide a concrete and tangible way to begin to understand what to actually *do* and *say* in a move towards helping staff experience being more Person-Centred. In this way staff can achieve a basic level of understanding and skill in using contact work and begin to incorporate these in their daily caring role (Smith, 2011).

Contact work

The development of contact is facilitated by the worker reflecting and mirroring – these are called *contact reflections*. Small behaviours from the client indicate flickers of response to the contact reflections – called *contact behaviours*. The contact reflections are summarised below with notes on their use with people with dementia. The dialogue below illustrates these contact reflections and behaviours with a resident with a severe level of dementia.

Contact reflections

Word-for-Word Reflections (WWR): Repeating words, phrases or words which seem to have importance or significance. This includes repeating and reflecting back sounds and utterances. The worker suspends their own understanding of words, as they may have particular meaning to a person with dementia. The worker follows the language pattern of the person with dementia. This may also include mirroring the tone, intonation and rhythm of any utterances.

Facial Reflections (FR): Mirroring back both verbally and non-verbally the facial expression or movements of the person with dementia. This is done sensitively, subtly and empathically in order to not appear mocking or disrespectful.

Bodily Reflections (BR): The movements, gestures, posture and motion of the person with dementia is reflected back. Again this may be verbally or non-verbally with non-verbal reflections often strengthening verbal reflections.

Situational Reflections (SR): The worker offers reflections about the surrounding environment – sounds, sights, location. Care is needed to limit imposing a reality that may not be shared by the person with dementia. For example, they may believe that they are on a ship instead of being in a room, a magazine may be a pack of important documents.

Reiterative Reflections (RR): Given the difficulty with memory, reiteration is more frequently in the moment. Contact reflections which appear to have elicited a response would be repeated or noted and the worker may reinforce this by drawing attention to an exchange which held greater contact.

An example of dialogue using contact reflections and contact behaviours

> Resident and nurse are both seated. Nurse sits on the right of the resident.
>
> Resident: [Sits staring ahead, blinking slowly, small movements of her right hand.]
>
> Nurse: You're sitting with your legs crossed (BR), your eyes look ahead. (FR) [The nurse mirrors the body posture.]
>
> Resident: [No response.]
>
> Nurse: You tap. [Nurse mirrors the movement of the right hand with her left hand which is closer to the resident.]
>
> [The nurse maintains the same pace as the resident.]
>
> Resident: [Stops tapping – this may be a contact behaviour as the client may have become aware of their own tapping.]
>
> Nurse: [Stops tapping.]
>
> Resident: Too who ... it's ... it's ...
>
> Nurse: To who.
>
> Resident: Tooooo who ... [The resident's facial expression changes to hold more intensity, still looking ahead.] [There may be contact developing here as the resident repeats the word 'Too' but gives more emphasis as if conveying its importance to the nurse.]
>
> Nurse: You look ahead. (FR)
>
> Resident: It's near there and where do well. [Resident leans forward and right hand moves as if to try and grasp something.]
>
> Nurse: You say 'too who' and look ahead (RR) and you reach out with your hand. (BR) [Nurse also reaches out with hand nearest resident and mirrors the movement.]
>
> Resident: [Touches the nurse's outstretched hand with theirs (contact behaviour) and says:] Yes who.
>
> Nurse: We touch and you say 'who'. (RR)
>
> Resident: [Resident holds the nurses wrist and strokes it with the other hand and their face and body posture become more relaxed. (contact behaviour)]

Working with people whose level of dementia is severe means that we may never know or understand what they are experiencing. However, people show increased signs of contact in the three domains described by Prouty et al. (2002): reality contact (i.e., contact with the surroundings or the world around them), affective contact (i.e., contact with their own experience of themselves), and communicative contact (i.e., the expression of the person's experience in the world, experience of themselves and conveying this to others through language or movement).

Reality contact

Mr X is staring at a plate of food. He holds a fork in his hand. It is not clear whether he recognises the fork and plate as food and Mr X needs help and prompting to eat. He is able to use cutlery but needs help establishing this action.

> Nurse: The plate is there (SR), green peas (SR) and your hand with a fork. (BR)
>
> Mr X: [Touches the fork with the other hand. (reality contact)]
>
> Nurse: The peas are green. (SR)
>
> Mr X: [Touches the peas with his empty hand, trying to pick them up. (reality contact)]
>
> Nurse: [Stays still.]
>
> Mr X: [Uses both fork and hand to eat peas – reality contact strengthened sufficiently for Mr X to start eating independently.]

Affective contact

Mrs A stands by the door of the hospital ward. Her face is angry; her body posture is tense and hostile. Her breathing is rapid and her words are disjointed. She has a pattern of becoming more agitated in the late afternoon.

> Mrs A: ... don't tell me you can't find them too ... it's all wrong from around here ... and help me towards it NOW you hear ...
>
> Nurse: You stand by the door (SR), and your breathing is fast (BR). [Nurse mirrors the posture of Mrs A's shoulders and the nurse holds her hand to her chest, breathing fast. (BR)]
>
> Mrs A: Yes and you can get on with it too, there's no to ... no help.
>
> Nurse: No one to help. (WWR) [Nurse very subtly mirrors her facial expression which appears to be fear and anguish. (FR)]
>
> Mrs A: No one, there's no one here. (Affective contact)

Communicative contact

Mr J has been repeatedly standing by a window where there is a bowl of plastic flowers. Several times members of staff have made conversational comments such as 'those look lovely' or 'do you like flowers'. These conversational openings do not usually develop any further than Mr J turning to look at the person who made the comment. The use of contact reflections illustrates a different approach and illustrates Mr J showing communicative contact.

> Mr J stands by the window sill in front of the flowers. Penny approaches:
>
> Penny: You stand by the window.
>
> Mr J: [No response.]
>
> Penny: The flowers are there. (SR) [Nurse points to the flowers.]
>
> Mr J: [Looking at the flowers and reaches to touch them. (showing reality contact)]
>
> Penny: [Stays silent.]
>
> Mr J: [Continues to look at flowers, shifting weight from foot to foot slightly.]
>
> Penny: You look at the flowers and move your legs. (SR, BR)
>
> Mr J: My wife.
>
> Penny: Your wife. (WWR)
>
> Mr J: My wife.
>
> Penny: You look at the flowers and say, 'my wife'. (SR, RR)
>
> Mr J: The crematorium. (Communicative contact)

Pre-Therapy in a dementia care context

A number of challenges face us when using contact work with people with severe dementia: Person-Centred care alongside practical and physical care; gauging expressiveness; the different experiences of reality of staff and people with dementia; the care context, and the emotional labour for staff.

Person-Centred care alongside practical and physical care

Whilst a principle of Person-Centred Therapy is attention to the immediate phenomenal world of the person, the reality of caring for people in later stages of dementia is that staff frequently do have to assume responsibility for ensuring that people receive help with activities and functions that they can no longer perform independently such as helping people wash, find their way around, eat.

Contact work lends itself to helping people in practical ways with their everyday care. The following excerpt is taken from the third of eleven sessions using Pre-Therapy with a woman with dementia – Joyce. Staff reported that she had not spoken in two years and generally avoided all contact with staff by walking away or looking at the floor. Staff described her as appearing expressionless or angry. She regularly refused food or drink given directly to her.

> Joyce is seated in the lounge with her head down and hands folded under her chin. Emma, the psychology trainee enters the room.

Emma: Hello Joyce, the sun is shining outside today. (SR)

Joyce: [Joyce lifts her head, then folds her hands back under her chin and looks at the floor again.]

Emma: Your head is looking down and you've got your hands folded under your chin.

[Therapist mirrors Joyce's body position. (BR)]

[Therapist and client remain like this for a few moments.]

Emma: Your cardigan is blue. It matches the colour of your eyes Joyce. (SR)

Joyce: [Joyce looks up and then gets out of her chair and starts to walk along the corridor.]

Emma: I hope you don't mind, but I am going to join you walking along the corridor.

Joyce: [Joyce looks up at the therapist then back to the floor and continues to walk.]

Emma: You are walking along the corridor Joyce and you are looking at the floor. (SR, BR)

Joyce: [Joyce walks slightly ahead of the therapist and looks back, and then at the floor, then looks back at the therapist before continuing to walk.]

[Therapist and client walk around the ward for a few minutes.]

Emma: You are walking past your bedroom Joyce. (SR)

Joyce: I don't want to go to bed.

Emma: You don't want to go to bed Joyce. (WRR)

Joyce: [Joyce runs her hands through her hair and looks anxious.]

Emma: You run your hands through your hair, and you look anxious.

[Therapist runs her hands through her hair. (FR, BR)]

[Therapist and client continue to walk quietly for a few moments.]

Emma: You walked along the corridor and you walked past your bedroom and you said 'I don't want to go to bed'. (RR)

Joyce: [Joyce looks up and smiles at the therapist.]

Emma: [Therapist smiles] You are smiling at me. (BR, FR)

[Joyce walks into the lounge and therapist follows. Joyce sits down, folds her hands under her chin and looks down at the floor. The therapist sits next to her; a tea trolley is wheeled in.]

Emma: The tea trolley is here and everyone is having a cup of tea. Would you like one Joyce? (SR)

Joyce: [Looks up and then runs her hands through her hair.]

Emma: You look anxious as you run your hands through your hair. [Therapist mirrors. (BR)]

[Therapist picks up a cup of tea and offers it to Joyce.]

Joyce: [Looks up, accepts the tea and drinks.]

Emma: We are sitting together and you are drinking a cup of tea. (SR)

Joyce: [Looks at therapist and drinks her tea.]

Gauging expressiveness

The theory of Pre-Therapy rests on the concept of people being either *in contact* or *expressive,* or *out of contact (pre-expressive)*. Van Werde (2002) identifies a place where a client may appear to be drifting in and out of contact or that contact is weak – the 'grey zone'. In our experience people with dementia can oscillate rapidly between seeming to be pre-expressive and highly expressive. This can make it difficult to follow the client's experience and to gauge when to use Pre-Therapy contact work and when to offer a response which is not a contact reflection, rather, working with the contact that has been established to offer a conversational response, or a question, suggestion or another form of communication. It is not always clear whether a person is entirely in contact as the cognitive and neurological changes affecting language affect their ability to convey this. This may be the case with Mrs A who was angry by the door. In one sense her expression of emotion was clear from the outset, so arguably she was in touch with her experience. However, we could equally argue that the contact work allowed time and space for her to be able to more clearly experience and express this. Dodds' (2008) doctoral work showed that, at times, very rapid emotional contact was established between the worker and person with dementia which sometimes surprised staff and also led to staff being faced with quite raw emotional states.

Experiences of reality

Prouty is clear that reality is experienced in objective, subjective and temporal senses. The example of Mr J and the flowers illustrates a potential difficulty regarding the nature of the word 'reality'. People with dementia frequently experience or inhabit a different reality to the consensual reality of those around them who do not have a cognitive impairment. Our challenge is to remain respectful and open to the subjective and temporal reality of the client. Contact work allows the client to explore and expand their own sense of reality. This counteracts the danger of imposing the consensual reality on someone with dementia or a person who may be straddling or existing within different temporal realities, and allows their internal, subjective reality to be honoured. With the example of Mr J, we see that his experience of reality is that his thoughts and experience of sadness are associated with the death of his wife. The flowers act as a prompt to this. His subjective and temporal realities are different from the staff who previously engaged with him by trying to prompt a conversation based in their reality. Staff in residential contexts have to working amongst multiple concurrent realities – their own and the people with dementia. A rolled-up newspaper may, in the mind's eye of the person with dementia, be an important document. The cardigan of another resident may be the coat of their child who they cannot find. However, it is precisely the virtue of the contact reflections that they help us to continue to follow the world of the person and help guard against imposing our reality or ideas onto the experience of the person with dementia. They challenge ordinary habits and patterns of communicating with persons with dementia. Also, the use of vague pronouns such as 'it' and 'them', means that we lessen the use of specific language to allow the person with dementia to show us the way into their world.

The care context

Whilst there are challenges to using contact work in practice, they are practical reminders of exactly why it is important to strive to be Person-Centred. By adopting contact work we are encouraged to suspend our own interpretation of the world around us and allow the person with dementia to experience the world as they understand it and perhaps convey this to us so that we can understand their world.

If we fail to do this the person may recede from view. The extract below from Pam Bruce-Hay illustrates the importance of striving to continue to see the person and the potential consequences of not seeing and allowing a person to be seen. It also illustrates the challenge of using contact work in a communal space.

George had spent a week staying at a dementia respite unit – a temporary stay. On the morning he was due to be discharged to a care home in another town, he had been lying (unhurt) in his pyjamas, on the floor of one of the corridors alongside the bedrooms. He had refused all offers of food and drink, and declined to communicate with staff. A request for a psychiatric assessment was being considered as there was concern around his capacity to make decisions.

The dialogue took place over a number of hours.

> Pam: Hello, I have come to keep you company.
>
> [No response, George is lying on his side in his pyjamas.]
>
> Pam: You are lying on the floor in your pyjamas.
>
> [No response – George remains still. I lie down on the floor on my side facing him.]
>
> Pam: I am lying on the floor next to you.
>
> [No response.]
>
> Pam: You are lying on the floor, in the corridor and you only have your pyjamas on. [At this point I gently touch George's arm.]
>
> Pam: Your hand is cold.
>
> George: Don't touch me.
>
> Pam: I am sorry – you don't want me to touch you.
>
> George: You talk too much, don't talk to me.
>
> Pam: I talk too much, I am a chatterbox, and you don't want me to talk to you – but you are lying on the floor in your pyjamas and you are cold. [I risked touching his hand again.]
>
> George: I told you not to talk to me and don't touch me.

Pam: You told me not to talk to you but I keep talking.

[George turns on to his back.]

Pam: You are lying on your back ... this floor is very hard.

[A nurse brings us a glass of milk and a cup of tea. She chats to George, he does not speak. She fetches a blanket and tries to cover him, he throws it off. After about one-and-a-half hours together on the floor, I continued to use reflection and a variety of dialogue to try and understand the significance of his behaviour. I also sipped my tea whilst George declined to drink his milk.

At times, we were observed by other people who were curious, but said nothing. They politely moved away at my request, however, when I informed George that I had sent the curious observers away he seemed suspicious, that I was conspiring with them against him. I felt that this was progress – George had spoken to me spontaneously. However, I chose not to reflect this statement, choosing instead to reassure him using reiterative contact reflection.]

Pam: The people watching were wondering why we were lying on the floor. It is nothing to do with them and I have closed the doors.

George: I don't believe you; you are in it with them.

[A social worker comes to assess George and to explain his rights during this situation. George did not speak. The social worker informed him that two psychiatrists would be coming to speak to him. He seemed interested, although said nothing. Two hours had passed. I tried to mirror his position, and decided to take a risk.]

Pam: George, two psychiatrists are coming to talk to you; if they find you lying on the floor in your pyjamas, they might think you are mad.

[At this, George sat up, drank some milk and said to me:]

George: Take me to my bedroom.

[Accepting my help, he walked to the adjacent bedroom and got into bed. He drank more milk and accepted some sandwiches. When the psychiatrists came into his room, he asked if I would stay with him. When interviewed by the psychiatrists, he seemed able to fully engage, explaining his reasons for lying on the floor and finally accepting the idea of leaving the unit and moving to a residential home.

During the evening, George again made his protest and lay on the floor. A nurse lay on the floor beside him until he went back to bed. The following day he seemed quite calm and cheerful and left the unit, accompanied by the social worker. It has been reported that George seems to have settled into his new home.]

Our final challenges in using contact work and being Person-Centred with people with dementia are around the concept of emotional labour, the context in which care is delivered and the dependency and vulnerability associated with a dementing illness.

Emotional labour

As already stated, the majority of frontline care is not delivered by people who are schooled in Person-Centred Therapy. Rather, care is delivered by a relatively unqualified, poorly paid workforce (Hussain & Manthorpe, 2012). The low status of the position of the older person with dementia is reflected in the workforce who in turn may internalise the negative concept of the nature of the work and may themselves be disempowered within the care system (Brooker, 2007). The nature of care work means that the lived experience of staff may be one of feeling overwhelmed with the sheer quantity of physical tasks to do, the experience of not having enough time and not feeling able to know how to manage people who may exhibit some very challenging behaviour.

For example, Mrs A, who becomes agitated in the late afternoon, frequently will shout and call out. She will walk up and down the ward and cannot be distracted. Attempts to engage her in activities or other topics of conversation have minimal success. She becomes short tempered with other residents and has hit and pushed other people with dementia. One member of staff is needed to constantly observe her when she poses a risk to other people.

There are drives to increase core skills and competencies of frontline staff. Person-centred care principles underpin this: principles of seeing the individual and respecting and maintaining dignity, communicating effectively and creating opportunities to enhance the wellbeing and quality of life of people with dementia. However, it remains a challenge to ask staff to communicate in ways which may not feel 'natural' or which may be considered at odds with care practices of doing things *for* people, attending to physical care and tasks within a context where there is overwhelming unmet need from people with dementia.

Contact work sometimes facilitates rapid and emotive changes with people experiencing raw emotional states. Contact work and other Person-Centred approaches demand the capacity to be present for the person, to be open to their experience and to be offering intent to see, hear and understand. Whereas a psychotherapy session is conducted one-to-one for 50 minutes, the institutional milieu for people with dementia in residential settings means that we encounter environments which may be brimming with such raw emotions as despair, distress, horror, sadness, fear. Positive emotional states may co-exist but are less prominent. To engage with this milieu at length without a break is difficult to say the least, and emotional responses of staff may include feeling inadequate and guilty (Theodosius, 2008). Indeed, there is an argument that staff cannot sufficiently attend to their own emotional needs and that being emotionally disengaged is a natural defence against this anxiety (Dartington, 2007). It is this tension between promoting the use of contact work and acknowledgement of the difficulties which raises the question of what level of compassion and empathy it is reasonable to expect.

Conclusion

We see Prouty's work offering the following:

1. An identifiable way of working with people with moderate and severe dementia which is Person-Centred in theoretical and philosophical origins.

2. An approach which, due to the concrete and tangible nature of the contact reflections, helps staff experience and embody what it means to work from the clients' experience of the world. This holds the potential to move closer towards Person-Centred day-to-day care.

3. An approach which exists amongst other Person-Centred and person-centred practices and may offer a bridge between them.

Contact work helps put Person-Centred practice at the heart of everyday person-centred care and as people's dementia progresses there is a moral imperative that care does continue to address emotional and psychological needs. All too frequently care becomes task oriented and physically focused. There is a danger that the person with dementia may become remote and we need emotion-oriented work to help staff sustain a sense of continuing to see the person alongside the dementia. The concrete and tangible nature of the contact work means that it holds the potential to be understood and used by staff who may have little grounding in Person-Centred theory and practice. For staff whose learning style may be practical rather than academic, this practical way in to how to be more Person-Centred may help open the door further to person-centred care which is more strongly based on a Person-Centred approach. The context and the environment will continue to challenge staff and the capacity for Person-Centred practice; however we remain optimistic that the use of light touch contact work which is integrated into everyday care is possible.

All three of us strive to work in a way which is informed by Person-Centred theory and see this as a precursor to engagement. However, the nature of our client group requires us to use a range of approaches, and be fluid in transitioning between being Person-Centred and using person-centred approaches. What Pre-Therapy offers us is both an approach to engagement and explicit ideas about how to try and maintain contact, which in turn assists in the rapport with people and our capacity to be open to their world.

If, as we suggest, contact work was seen as part of everyday interaction, much as the glue holding pieces of mosaic together, then there is the potential to strengthen the capacity to hold the person central in all aspects of care. As dementia progresses, people show increasing difficulty in understanding the world around them, have problems communicating and present to us fragments of personal experiences which are difficult to understand. In this situation we need as many ways of engaging which help us try to be alongside them and their dementia in ways which hold and respect their own sense of personhood. Pre-Therapy offers a stepping stone to more depth where possible, and an engagement strategy that can later include other approaches.

The moral and ethical imperative to maintain a position of respect is inherent in person-centred dementia care. Dementia offers a challenge to the expression of self and one's personhood. It may become more difficult for people to assert their own self on the world, people may forget their names but still possess a sense of self and past selves, but the wider social world holds the danger of seeing an illness, not a person (Sabat, 2001). While people with dementia suffer many losses in function and capacity, they do not lose their essential humanity, and it is the sharing of common humanity that ensures their moral status.

> The core concern of ethics then, is the deep affirmation of common humanity and there is no reason to exclude anyone from that affirmation, based on the mere fact that they have become more deeply forgetful than the rest of us. (Post, 2006, p. 223)

By being open to the world dementia sufferers inhabit – that is, seeing them, understanding them and validating them – they can be enabled to feel alive, grounded and in touch with their experience and relate to their inner world and the world around them in the most meaningful way and to the fullest extent possible. Working therapeutically in relationships with people experiencing different stages of dementia means trying to preserve their sense of identity or personhood. Person-Centred practice offers listening to their narrative (however muddled) and engaging, whilst attempting to understand the deep, emotional significance of fragments of shared information or 'remnants' of their personal history and personal relationships. By offering undivided attention and emotional presence to share their silence and hold whatever their dialogue may contain, we believe it possible to facilitate the positive process and development of a person with dementia. This enables the person to optimise their personal resources for coping and making changes as they adjust to their experience of their illness.

Despite the pressures exerted by forces which label and dehumanise people with dementia and institutional arrangements which may hinder staff from being able to be human alongside humans with dementia we are hopeful for the place of Person-Centred practice in dementia care and the potential to facilitate people with dementia being able to experience ordinariness and normality in response to their very extraordinary situation.

> If we pass by the person with dementia just once and reach superficial conclusions, we fail morally. When we pass by a second time and begin to observe the complexity of a life lived in deep forgetfulness, respect becomes possible. (Post, 2006, p. 233)

References

Brooker, D (2007) *Person-Centred Dementia Care: Making services better.* London: Jessica Kingsley.

Brooker, D & Surr, C (2005) *Dementia Care Mapping: Principles and practice.* Bradford: Bradford Dementia Group.

Cheston, R (1998) Psychotherapeutic work with dementia sufferers. *Social Work Practice, 12*(2), 199–207.

Dartington, A (2007) Where angels fear to tread: Idealism, despondency and inhibition in thought in hospital nursing. In R Davenhill (Ed) *Looking into Later Life: A psychoanalytic approach to depression and dementia in old age* (pp. 160–85). London: Karnac Books.

Dodds, P (2008) Pre-Therapy and Dementia: An action research project. Unpublished PhD Thesis. University of Brighton.

Feil, N & De Klerk-Rubin, V (2012) *The Validation Breakthrough: Simple techniques for communicating with people with Alzheimer's type dementia* (3rd ed). Baltimore, MD: Health Professions Press.

Gendlin, ET (1973) Experiential psychotherapy. In R Corsini (Ed) *Current Psychotherapies* (pp. 312–52). Itasca, IL: FE Peacock.

Greenwood, D (2007) Relational care: Learning to look beyond intentionality to the 'non-intentional' in a caring relationship. *Nursing Philosophy, 8*(4), 223–32.

Hussain, S & Manthorpe, J (2012) The dementia social care workforce in England: Secondary analysis of a national workforce dataset. *Aging and Mental Health, 16*(1), 110–18.

Kitwood, T (1997) *Dementia Reconsidered: The person comes first.* Buckingham: Open University Press.

McCance, T, McCormack, B & Dewing, J (2011) An exploration of person-centredness in practice. *OJIN: The Online Journal of Issues in Nursing, 16*(2), Manuscript 1. (May 31, 2011).

McCormack, B, Dewing. J & McCance, T (2011) Developing person-centred care: Addressing contextual challenges through practice development. *OJIN: The Online Journal of Issues in Nursing, 16*(2), Manuscript 3. (May 31, 2011).

Merleau-Ponty, M (2002) *Phenomenology of Perception: An introduction* (2nd rev ed). London: Taylor & Francis.

Post, S (2006) *Respectare:* Moral respect for the lives of the deeply forgetful. In JC Hughes, SJ Louw & SR Sabat (Eds) *Dementia: Mind, meaning, and the person* (pp. 223–34). Oxford: Oxford University Press.

Prouty, G (Ed) (2008) *Emerging Developments in Pre-Therapy: A Pre-Therapy reader.* Ross-on-Wye: PCCS Books.

Prouty, G, Van Werde, D & Pörtner, M (2002) *Pre-Therapy: Reaching contact-impaired clients.* Ross-on-Wye: PCCS Books.

Rogers, CR (1951) *Client-Centered Therapy.* Boston: Houghton Mifflin.

Rogers, CR (1959) A theory of therapy, personality and interpersonal relationships, as developed in the client-centered framework. In S Koch (Ed) *Psychology: A study of science, Vol. 3: Formulations of the person and the social context* (pp. 184–256). New York: McGraw-Hill.

Sabat, S (2001) *The Experience of Alzheimer's Disease: Life through a tangled veil.* Oxford: Blackwell.

Sanders, P (Ed) (2007) *The Contact Work Primer.* Ross-on-Wye: PCCS Books.

Smith, P (2011) Using Pre-Therapy to release long silent voices. *Journal of Dementia Care.* 19(5), 20–2.

Theodosius, C (2008) *Emotional Labour in Nursing: The unmanaged heart of nursing*. Abingdon: Routledge.

Van Werde, D (2002) A contact milieu. In G Prouty, D Van Werde and M Pörtner (Eds) *Pre-Therapy: Reaching contact-impaired clients* (pp. 77–114). Ross-on-Wye: PCCS Books.

Van Werde, D & Morton, I (1999) The relevance of Prouty's Pre-Therapy to dementia care. In I Morton (Ed) *Person-Centred Approaches to Dementia Care* (pp. 139–66). Bicester: Winslow Press.

Van Werde, D & Prouty, G (2013) Clients with contact-impaired functioning: Pre-Therapy. In M Cooper, M O'Hara, PF Schmid & AC Bohart (Eds) *The Handbook of Person-Centred Counselling and Psychotherapy* (2nd ed, pp. 327–43). Basingstoke: Palgrave Macmillan.

Part 2
Conceptualisations that support practice

Client processes at the difficult edge | 10

Margaret Warner

Carl Rogers (1957) proposes that client-centred therapy[1] is 'necessary and sufficient' to bring constructive personality change to clients at *all levels of distress or dysfunction*. Rogers asserts that this therapy – characterised by empathy, genuineness, and unconditional positive regard – does not need outside interpretation, confrontation, or structured interventions to be effective. In fact, the theory proposes that such interventions often interfere with the client's self-directed process and choice.

The 'difficult process' model of client-centred psychotherapy that I am presenting in this chapter does not challenge Rogers' core approach to psychotherapy, i.e., his proposition that the six well-known conditions are 'necessary and sufficient' to produce change in the absence of any structured intervention, interpretation or confrontation. In fact, I find that the essential non-directivity of a classically oriented client-centred psychotherapy is often particularly helpful to clients experiencing severe distress and dysfunction (see also Sommerbeck, Chapter 12, this volume).

The difficult process model does, however, aim to provide a useful addition to Rogers' theory in two ways. First, I believe that the effectiveness of person-centred psychotherapy with severe client distress and dysfunction is better *explained* if person-centred developmental theory is expanded by not only considering conditions of worth, but also (a) the development of processing capacities within the early attachment relationships of infancy, (b) the development of self-cohesion within such early attachment relationships, and (c) the overall self-healing capacities of the brain (see also Peters, Chapter 11, this volume). Second, client-centred therapists may be better able to *understand* their clients and to *convey their understanding* in ways that clients can receive when they are familiar with common experiences of difficult process and difficult self.

---

1. The classical, non-directive form of Rogerian therapy tends to be called 'client-centred' in Chicago, but person-centred in many other parts of the world. I am keeping to the Chicago usage of the words 'client-centred' in this chapter, and using 'person-centred' to refer to Rogers' overall theory and the broader range of therapies based in his approach.

In my work, I have become familiar with three particular kinds of process – 'fragile process', 'dissociated process' and 'psychotic process' – which are often experienced as exceedingly difficult by clients and/or therapists. (I am sure that others could be delineated.) Stated very briefly, fragile process occurs when clients have difficulty holding core experiences in attention at moderate levels of intensity and have difficulty taking in viewpoints outside of their frames of reference without feeling that their own experience has been annihilated; dissociated process occurs when clients hold experience within separate, quasi-autonomous 'selves' or 'parts'. Psychotic process occurs when clients' experiences and expressions are difficult to understand and are outside of ordinary norms of expression. In addition to difficult forms of process, I have also begun to consider the ways that difficult experiences of *self* are often (but not always) paired with experiences of difficult process. I will describe these difficult forms of process and self in greater depth later in this chapter.

I want to emphasise that these categories of 'difficult process' and 'difficult self' are descriptions of some common client experiences rather than diagnostic categories. They are useful to person-centred therapists to the degree that they help therapists understand and to convey their understanding to their clients and to maintain their sense of unconditional positive regard and genuineness within the relationship. Let us begin by considering developmental issues in relation to Rogers' original person-centred theory.

Rogers' personality theory

Rogers' (1951, 1959) personality theory suggests that individuals tend to inhibit their abilities to process experience when they have conditions of worth which have been conveyed to them by significant others, especially the primary caregivers of childhood. These conditions of worth are transmitted as significant others withdraw their positive regard in response to particular ways of being that the child may manifest. In other words a 'condition of worth' is a particularly strong sort of attitude or value which has been internalised.

Still, the consideration of conditions of worth alone does not provide a strong explanation as to why person-centred therapy should work with many more severe forms of psychological distress and dysfunction. Biological damage to the brain (and the whole physiological organism that participates in brain functioning) is not in and of itself a manifestation of the sorts of internalised attitudes conceptualised by Rogers as 'conditions of worth'. Yet such biological difficulties are likely to be involved in many severe forms of psychological distress and dysfunction – such as traumatic brain injury, dementia and some forms of psychosis.

One major expansion of theory that I am proposing involves including the development of processing *capacities* as they develop with early infant attachment.

I am referring to 'process' or processing, in the common person-centred usage, referring to the sorts of changes that experience often goes through when attended to with an accepting attitude.

Attachment relationships in infancy

The concept of attachment was developed by Bowlby (1969, 1988) and elaborated by others such as Mahler, Pine and Bergman (1975) to describe dyadic relationships between infant and caregiver allowing mutually pleasurable interaction and increasingly autonomous exploration by the infant in the context of a secure relationship with the caregiver. Substantial research has documented the ongoing impact of such attachment styles later in life (Main, 1991; Schore, 2003).

From a person-centred point of view, the attachment relationship can be seen as an early, characteristically human form of actualisation. Infants and their caregivers have a natural inclination to develop stable forms of relating and to simultaneously develop the capacities necessary to process experience. Ideally these capacities develop within secure attachment relationships in early childhood. But, I (and others) propose that the inherent developmental tendency remains throughout life, and can be picked up later within relationships that have some of the qualities of safety, connection and empathic attunement that is characteristic of such early attachment relationships (Kohut, 1971, 1984; Lee & Martin, 1991; Warner, 1997, 2000; Vanaerschot, 2004).

Development of processing capacities within attachment relationships

Safety and care

Infants are almost completely reliant on their caregivers to moderate the intensity of their experience. If adults are unable or unwilling to provide care, infants are flooded with experience in ways that are akin to torture. Such experiences can easily create a deeply held belief that bodily experience is a bad thing, best ignored.

Holding experience in attention

Infants on their own don't maintain a sustained focus of attention. Without adult engagement, they easily become bored and cranky. Mutually pleasurable non-verbal and verbal interactions not only create pleasurable relationship experiences, they develop the brain's ability to focus attention. Such focused interchanges seem tied to the level of attunement of the caregiver.

Numerous studies have found that mothers of infants who become securely attached show high levels of moment-to-moment attunement both in initiating interactions and in responding to distress (Sroufe, 1996, pp. 166–8, 185–88).

Modulating the intensity of experience

Based on studies of heart rate and gaze aversion, Fogel (1982) finds that over the first year of life, secure infants gradually become able to moderate levels of arousal while staying engaged in pleasurable interactions with caregivers for longer periods of time. Less securely attached infants seem to come to a different set of capacities and beliefs. They find (1) that it is difficult to maintain emotionally engaged attention in a way that leads to sustained positive experiences, (2) that situations of high arousal are likely to lead to overload and disorganisation and (3) caregivers aren't very effective in soothing distress when it does occur.

Naming experience

Areas of the brain central to logical and verbal processing mature later in infancy and early childhood. Certainly, conditions of worth are likely to play a part in determining what sorts of experience can be comfortably named within a particular family; in a relatively secure environment, there is room for children to remain aware of their visceral experience when naming what they are feeling. They are able to moderate the intensity of their reactions enough that they can hold their experience in attention.

Combined together, these capacities developed within secure attachment relationships allow what Mary Main (1991, p. 128) calls 'metacognitive' functioning. This capacity allows individuals to attend to and resolve contradictions in their experiences generating a single, reasonably integrated, narrative organising their life experience, what Rogers would call a 'congruent' sense of self.

Fragile self and the development of self in infancy

Rogers' theory of self suggests that difficulties arise when there is an incongruence between experiences held within the self and experiences which arise from the totality of the person's organism. Under these circumstances, the experiences of the organism are not well symbolised in awareness. So, for example, if I think of myself as a generous person, but find myself wanting to keep something for myself rather than giving to someone else who really needs it, I may experience a great deal of anxiety because of the contradiction between self and organism.

Heinz Kohut (1971, 1984) conceptualises another quality of self, namely, 'cohesiveness', which I think can be a useful addition to the person-centred understanding of self without taking anything away from Rogers' initial conceptualisation. Kohut notes that infants are heavily reliant on caregivers to maintain a sense of emotional balance and wellbeing. He calls this (with a typically psychoanalytic denseness of language) a 'selfobject' relationship. Kohut's selfobject relationship closely parallels the 'securely attached' infant relationships described by the developmental psychologists cited earlier.

Kohut suggests that given good-enough selfobject relationships in infancy, a person will develop a relatively independent capacity for maintaining emotional balance and sense of self-worth. Without a cohesive sense of self, as Kohut calls it, a person is likely to experience a great deal of volatility in adulthood. Often such a person will seek out highly supportive, dependent selfobject relationships in adulthood to maintain emotional balance. This strategy often works quite well as long as that relationship continues without disruption. However, even a small misunderstanding can create a rupture in the relationship. Then, a person is likely to experience extreme distress, volatility, and felt worthlessness – a state Kohut calls 'fragmentation'. In response to these extreme feelings, people often engage in a variety of behaviours that cause difficulties – such as self-harm, vengeful behaviour and demeaning communication. They often threaten to cut off previously valued selfobject relationships.

Kohut (1971, 1984) proposes that a stable, empathic, non-interpretive therapy can allow a client to use the therapist as a selfobject, re-initiating the developmental process that was missing or disrupted in childhood. Certainly, client-centred therapy seems ideally suited to this situation. In such relationships the client can gradually develop a cohesive sense of self. The self, then, can be viewed as a human phenomenon that not only provides coherence (or congruence in Rogers' terms) but also helps a person modulate emotional intensity and to maintain a sense of personal existence and value.

Processing capacities and the brain

Of course, the capacities of processing and self listed above – and many other capacities that undergird human functioning – require a normatively functioning brain. These capacities can be interfered with by genetic or perinatal difficulties, brain damage or brain degeneration. I will not be addressing these brain issues in any depth in this chapter other than to suggest the following core hypotheses: Processing capacities are essential to effective human functioning, in that they are essential to the creation of meaning. Like many other such capacities that are essential to human survival, they are over-determined within the human organism. The human brain has a number of alternative pathways to processing, each with its distinctive strengths and weaknesses. When brain capacities relating to processing are disrupted, human beings will continue to try to process with those capacities remaining. These ways of processing may *sound* very different from more normative expressions, but they allow significant processing to happen and have a major impact on the client's sense of personal meaning, relationship and overall wellbeing.

Recent scientific work has found much more plasticity to the brain and ability to recover lost functioning than was previously thought (Doidge, 2007). Connecting with the capacities that the person has in an atmosphere of safety allows discovery of alternative modes of processing. And it seems to stimulate regeneration of processing capacities to the extent that this is biologically possible.

This view of processing and brain function has considerable implication for person-centred theory and practice. Historically, many theorists have thought that psychotherapy was only effective as a response to issues grounded in clients' social and emotional histories as opposed to issues grounded in brain biology. Clients who were seen as incapable of 'insight' often were not offered counselling or psychotherapy at all. Instead, such clients were offered medication, social programming or fairly basic social skills training.

If, as I am proposing, the brain is inherently organised to try to process meaning, the differences between biological and socio-emotional genesis of problems become much less significant. For person-centred therapists, the same overall approach is likely to be helpful whether issues are biologically or psychologically based (or both).

With these additions to Rogers' core theory in mind, let us turn to considering each of the three forms of difficult process and self in greater depth.

Fragile process

Clients who experience fragile process (Warner, 1997, 2000, 2001) have difficulty holding experience in attention at moderate levels of intensity and, as a result, have difficulty starting and stopping experiences that are personally significant or emotionally connected. Such personal experiences are often sensed as shameful or likely to cause harm to the client or to others in relationship with the client. Because they have difficulty holding onto their own experience, clients often find that they have difficulty taking in the point of view of another person without feeling that their own experience has been annihilated.

Therapists often greatly underestimate how sensitive clients are when they are in the middle of fragile process. In general, client-centred therapists focus on empathic responding and avoid even moderately directive questions, suggestions or interpretations. Yet, at vulnerable moments a client may need even more precise forms of empathic understanding responses. The client may need to hear the therapist's understanding in almost his or her exact words to feel understood. Or, when a client is attending to something that is unclear, open-ended words like 'something' or 'somehow' may let the therapist 'make space' for the unclearness in what the client is saying without adding any contrary meaning. For example, a client may feel very touched when he or she feels understood by the therapist's close empathic responding:

> Cl: I feel a sinking, scared feeling about going to this job interview.
>
> Th: A sinking scared feeling ... Something about going to this job interview gives you a sinking scared feeling ...
>
> Cl: Yes, exactly. [Tears]

Yet, even quite close paraphrasing of a client's words may result in his or her losing the ability to hold the experience. This can lead to a feeling that the experience (and possibly her self in relation to the therapist) has been annihilated – leading the client to feel enraged or to give up on the interaction and withdraw. For example,

> Cl: I feel a sinking, scared feeling about going to this job interview ...
>
> Th: You're worried that this job interview isn't going to go well.
>
> Cl: I DIDN'T SAY THE INTERVIEW WASN'T GOING TO GO WELL!!! WHY DID YOU SAY THAT??? YOU DON'T UNDERSTAND ME AT ALL.

Even more so, therapist comments and questions that are intended to be helpful and to advance the client's self-exploration are likely to backfire. For example, the client may feel deeply wounded.

> Cl: You think my feelings are all wrong or you wouldn't have asked that question. Something is always wrong with me!! I think you have never respected me as a human being!!

The risk here is that therapists can easily see clients' anger or withdrawal as the client's problem – without seeing that the therapist's behaviour has a great deal to do with the client's response. Therapists assume that clients could turn off fragile process if they wanted to. They then proceed to view clients as tricky or manipulative.

Another sort of risk comes from therapists' personal reactions to clients, times when therapists lose congruence and their ability to trust the client's own process. This, of course, can happen in relation to any clients. But, in my experience clients in the midst of fragile process are particularly likely to evoke these sorts of incongruent therapist reactions since clients in the midst of fragile process often have a sort of tunnel vision in interpreting their own experience.

Take the following example:

> A woman's friend promised to come over to help her get her apartment ready for a party that was very important to her. The friend never came and didn't call. She was furious and hurt. The next day she called her friend and he apologised profusely. He said that his child had been taken to the

emergency room earlier in the afternoon and he had been so preoccupied
that he had forgotten that this was the day of the party.

Clients in the midst of fragile process sometimes find that it takes everything
that they have to stay connected with their own immediate experience – which is
often very intense and disturbing. So, their viewpoint at that time may be totally
tied to their own reactions with little attention to other elements of the context.
From this place a client might say: 'I should have known better than to think he
would come. People are only out for themselves', or 'I feel so hurt, I will never
again let myself think I can have anything special like a party just for myself'. Or
'He was never going to come. He just said that so that I would be humiliated in
front of all my colleagues.'

I have often found that as a therapist, I have strong impulses to bring in
other perspectives when clients speak in ways that seem to me to be extremely
one-sided or unrealistic or insensitive to other people in the client's life. At these
moments, I tend to feel that some small, common-sensical piece of insight or
advice will make the client's situation much easier. I find myself explaining:
'Having your child taken to the emergency room is likely to be very overwhelming;
I can understand someone really forgetting under those circumstances ...', or
reassuring: 'I think you can have wonderful parties in the future – this was just a
one-time difficulty because of your friend's emergency', or contradicting: 'I doubt
that he wanted you to feel humiliated ...'.

Two points are important here. First, I have found that when clients are in
the midst of fragile experiences, they seldom find these sorts of comments from
me to be illuminating. Rather, they have often responded by feeling that I have
just made their experience worthless and stupid. One client would often say
when I found myself making comments like the above: 'I thought that this would
be at least one place where I could feel understood'.

The second point is that when I do stay empathically connected with
clients in a personal process that seems one-sided to me, it does seem to help
clients both immediately and in the long run. In the short run, having a place to
have your experience honoured just as it is allows a person to be received as a
worthwhile human being, and this makes it much easier to cope with immediate
life circumstances. In the longer run, I find that the experience of person-centred
therapy offers a holding environment in which clients' process tends to pick up
its development where it left off earlier in life.

Work with fragile self

Clients may not only experience fragile process in a moment-to-moment way.
They may also experience a fragile self. One image that I have for this is that
of a rubber ball, which can be pressed out of shape with the confidence that
when the pressure is released it will return to its original shape. If people have

a cohesive sense of self, they may find themselves in the midst of experiences that are very strange or disturbing or contrary to the person they thought they were. Yet, they still have some feeling that their sense of a solid, (at least somewhat) worthwhile self will return over time. It may be altered, but it will not be destroyed or annihilated or made into something totally worthless. One might say that cohesiveness is a quality that allows a person to tolerate moderately high levels of experienced incongruence for a period of time. Without a certain level of cohesiveness, experiences of incongruence can be terrifying. It is not simply that I feel angry or upset or disturbed. I feel that these experiences are forever, leaving me with no sense of self and no human value.

A fragile sense of self can add greater intensity to a client's need to hold strongly to versions of their experience that have the sort of tunnel vision that I described above. If a client's formulation is seen to be *wrong*, it is not only that particular formulation that is at risk, but the person's whole self and the relationships the person is engaged in are at risk of being annihilated forever.

Like Kohut, person-centred therapists create stable, secure, empathic relationships that parallel those of healthy parent–infant attachment relationships. The relationship itself helps clients maintain much higher levels of emotional balance and sense of personal worth than they are able to without the relationship. And, the ongoing stability of these relationships allows a cohesive sense of self to develop over time. But, these relationships are easy to rupture, creating a sudden drastic change into volatility, panic and relationship cut-off as well as a variety of behaviours that function as attempts to get away from the terror of this experience. Kohut (1984) notes that ongoing, non-judgemental, empathic connection tends to allow the relationship to be restored. The non-directivity of classical client-centred therapy, then, makes this therapy particularly likely to be helpful to clients who struggle with living with a self that lacks cohesiveness.

Dissociated process and dissociated selves

Development of dissociated self and dissociated process

Clients' accounts of their dissociative experiences in combination with the general literature on dissociative identity disorders have allowed person-centred therapists to construct an understanding of the origin and functioning of trauma-driven dissociation.[2]

The clients we have seen who have experienced dissociative parts virtually all came to remember experiences of sexual or physical trauma before the age of 7. At

---

2. The overall understanding that person-centred theorists have of dissociative phenomena is quite similar to that of more directively oriented therapists, such as Kluft (1985), Putnam (1989), or Braun (1986). These phenomena do, however, present themselves in significantly different ways in a client-directed therapeutic process.

such early ages children have high levels of openness to imagination and hypnotic suggestibility. Faced with overwhelming trauma and lacking the more complex ways of coping with experiences available to older children, our clients seem to have stumbled on dissociation as a solution. One client, for example, found that when she stared at dots on the wallpaper she could separate herself out from the terror and anguish of being raped by her father. Some clients describe experiencing themselves as out of their bodies and watching the events from the ceiling.

Understandably, dissociation under these circumstances is extremely reinforcing. Children go from an overwhelming state of anguish to a lack of intense pain and an ability to put the whole thing out of their minds the next day. This capacity makes family life seem tolerable and, for some, allows the illusion that they have a normal, happy family life. Clients seem to take a larger lesson from the apparent effectiveness of these early experiences of dissociation – that emotional pain is destructive and that the way to live successfully is to make painful experiences disappear.

Such early childhood dissociation seldom seems to stop with amnesia or emotional separation from the experience within a unified personality, as is typical of adult posttraumatic stress disorders. Children almost always divide the dissociated aspects of their experiences into a number of compartments that are separate from each other. I suspect that this happens because young children have a number of intense reactions that seem irreconcilable with each other and they do not yet have the mental capacities to integrate such contradictions.

Probably as a result of these contradictions, a number of different clusters of experience were separated out within our clients' dissociated experiences. These clusters of experience came to have a very distinctive sort of *person-like* experience of themselves, each with its own feelings, history, and way of looking at the world. A number of dissociated parts typically take on self-abusive or suicidal qualities. These impulses seem to arise when the pain of dissociated memories threatens to return. Typically, though not always, this anguish is held by a young child part who is terrified and alone and wishes someone would come help. (Angry abusive parts are also frightened children and have their own disturbing memories that they may be trying to get away from.)

Dissociated process

Clients who experience dissociated process go through periods of time when they quite convincingly experience themselves as having selves that are not integrated with each other (Warner, 1998, 2000; Roy, 1991; Coffeng, 1996). Sometimes, they directly experience a disunity of self that feels disturbing to themselves and to others. For example, one client of mine could experience a girl child down to her left and a boy down to her right. Yet when she attended to those parts, actions that had been puzzling in the previous week often became clear. For example, she had torn up a year's work of artwork one week with no understanding of why she had done this. Yet, when she looked down at the boy part during the next session, she said, '*He* did it. He's angry about the things I talked about last week ….'.

At other times clients may have periods of forgetfulness for the minutes or hours when alternate personality parts have been dominant. A client may say, 'I really don't remember much about the hour when I was in my boss's office. I know he started criticising me in a very demeaning way, but I don't remember much after that ….' Or, clients may find themselves taking actions that are congruent with dissociated parts but highly incongruent with their everyday sense of themselves or their intentions. For example, one client from the Counseling Center, who was a very kind person in general, found herself tripping people on the street with no sense of why that was happening. Later, a part emerged in the client's therapy who said, 'Sure I tripped them. And I'm not sorry. No one should get away with treating children the way those people did ….'

Clients may go for years without being aware of such parts by keeping very busy and leading quite restricted lives, only to have such 'crazy-feeling' parts or parts-related experiences emerge in times of crisis. At this point clients (as well as mental health professionals) can easily see them as being in the midst of a severe psychotic break, sometimes wondering if this is the beginning of a life-long struggle with schizophrenia.

Dissociated self

Clients in a higher-functioning aspect of themselves may have quite normative ideas about what is real and sensible. Yet, when a part has taken over, that part may have some ideas that seem irrational to outsiders and to the client herself in her everyday awareness. They may:

- see things that are not there, as when a male part looks in the mirror and sees himself as male, when the client is female.

- believe things that the client in her everyday self would find unreasonable. For example, a part said that he would like to slit the wrists of a girl part, but didn't think that he would be harmed in the process.

- have physiological reactions that are related to parts' experiences – such as having different allergies or different eyesight, or different reading abilities when a part has taken over.

Person-centred therapy with dissociated self and process

Of course, all of these parts' experiences affect the therapeutic relationship. A client-centred therapist needs to take parts on their own terms, understanding that ideas about reality may shift rapidly as different parts take the centre of consciousness. A therapist's unconditional positive regard can't be reserved for some parts over others. For example, the part that wants to cut is as much a client as the part that is afraid of being cut. This is all the more challenging because parts themselves don't always think that other parts have the right to exist. The therapy, then, becomes more like family therapy than individual therapy in some ways, with the therapist holding the core conditions toward several quite different persons at once. The therapist can't assume that a trusting relationship with one part of the person extends to other parts of the person.

Person-centred therapy with dissociation differs from that of other orientations in the degree to which clients structure and guide the process. As a person-centred therapist, I don't try to get dissociated parts to come out. I don't try to stop them from coming. I just stay with the process as it emerges. Clients may deal with dissociated parts intensely for some period of time and then centre on more normative, higher-functioning parts of themselves for long periods of time. Yet parts tend to re-emerge in their own time, sometimes in response to a crisis, sometimes just as a part of the client's growth process.

When I am familiar and comfortable with these sorts of experiences, clients seem to feel safer engaging with those aspects of themselves. And, when clients ask, I am able to explain that I don't believe that these sorts of experiences imply any irreparable damage to the person; that they can be worked on in therapy very productively.

Psychotic process and psychotic self

When clients have a psychotic style of processing, their experience doesn't make sense within the culture and/or doesn't offer a predictive validity in relation to their environment. Such clients may experience voices, hallucinations or delusions that are neither culturally accepted nor easy to process (Prouty 1994, 2001; Prouty, Van Werde, & Pörtner, 2002). They may communicate in words and logics that seem bizarre or idiosyncratic to more normatively functioning people (Warner, 2002b; Warner & Trytten, 2008). Garry Prouty (1994, 2001) describes such clients as having impaired contact with 'self', 'world' and 'other'. Although Garry Prouty and I have some minor theoretical differences (Warner, 2002a), I follow Garry Prouty very closely in my understanding of psychotic process overall. Prouty notes that 'contact reflections' which are exceedingly close to clients' exact words and gestures often allow clients to develop psychological contact. And he observes that psychotic experiences are likely to process when therapists stay with them.

In my own paraphrased version, these contact reflections are:

1. *Word-for-word.* For example: Client: 'The gates aren't shutting right because of the devils in the east.' Th: 'Oh, I see. The gates really aren't shutting right because of the devils in the east.'

2. *Facial.* For example: The client is silent while tears stream down her face and she opens her mouth several times. Th: 'Tears are streaming down your face and you opened your mouth several times.'

3. *Bodily.* Clients may move without putting words to this. Therapists can make the same bodily motion or put it into words (or both). For example: The client makes a fist and hits the table; therapist makes a fist and hits the table and says: 'You made a fist and you hit the table!'

4. *Environmental.* Clients may attend to various things going on in the environment. For example: a truck goes by outside the therapy room and the client looks toward the sound. Th: 'A truck went by outside and you looked outside the window.'

5. *Reiterative.* Clients may say particularly striking and lucid things in the midst of process that is otherwise hard to follow. Therapists may return to those statements after a time. For example: Cl: 'My father really never wanted me to be born' followed by phrases that are hard to understand. Th: 'Your father really never wanted you to be born.'

As with fragile process, therapists often underestimate how close they need to stay with clients' concrete expressions for clients to know that they are being heard. For example, when I was first seeing my client 'Luke' I would often paraphrase his words in a way that seemed minor to me, and find that he did not know what I meant. For example, he might say 'I'm angry at the staff at my residence' and I might say 'You're really mad at them.' He, then, would say something like 'I don't know about "mad", doctor; but, you know more about these things than I do.'

In my own work, I have developed an understanding of a particular sort of psychotic experience, 'thought disorder' – which is common within schizophrenia and various sorts of dementia. I have found that thought disorder is a hybrid of ordinary logical/factual and ordinary metaphorical ways of experiencing. As such it is likely to sound very nonsensical. But I find that this sort of thought-disordered language processes in very productive ways (Warner (2002b; Warner & Trytten, 2008). One set of comments from Luke that I am quite fond of remembering went like this (slightly paraphrased, with metaphacts underlined):

> The trouble with the world is that there are too many Spaniards. My father is a Spaniard. When he talks, I only understand about a third of what he says. I think that that's because he comes from another country. On the other hand, you seem to understand me perfectly well. That must be because we come from the same country.

These comments *sound* as if Luke were speaking about clearly defined units (or facts) and clearly defined causal relations. After all, Luke observes that his father *is* a Spaniard and that his trouble understanding his father comes about *because* his father is from another country.

This is clearly not factual. Luke's father is an Irish American person and has never lived in another country to my knowledge.

Notably, Luke's whole train of thought – that seems so unreasonable when seen as a rendition of facts and causes – would make sense if it were reformulated in terms of the kinds of broad similarities characteristic of metaphors or similes rather than facts and causes. Thus, a person might quite sensibly say:

> The trouble in the world is that too many people <u>behave as if they were</u> Spaniards. They are proud and demanding and autocratic. I feel <u>as if</u> my father is like that. He <u>seems as if</u> he comes from another country. He <u>might as well</u> be speaking Spanish; I only understand about a third of what he says. Somehow, you and I <u>seem like</u> we come from the same country. You seem to understand me perfectly well.

As we can see here, metaphacts really are a hybrid of more ordinary facts and more ordinary metaphors. Luke doesn't seem to have the metaphoric distance that would let him clearly distinguish between figures of speech and literal facts. Yet, when Luke holds a metaphact image in mind, it tends to draw other related scenes, images and feelings to his mind, as would be typical when a higher-functioning client holds an image or metaphor relating to a complex life situation.

Several things are striking to me about Luke's process. When he ponders his life issues in metaphact language (as in the passage above), he tends to come to understandings that are quite sensible and normative in their broad outlines. After the processing in the passage above he might be more likely to say something about communication to his father or at least understand the source of his discomfort. Interestingly, he doesn't seem to hold onto the less sensible aspects of metaphacts as a factual reality over time. For example, he would not continue with the idea that his father was a Spaniard or think that he needed to learn Spanish to communicate with his father.

Luke himself doesn't find the metaphact language strange. When people comment on or try to correct his way of thinking or speaking he tends to just think that they are trying to hurt his feelings. Still, he does seem to know better than to speak in metaphact language very much in public. He calls this 'keeping his cards close to his chest …'.

My students' pilot research at the Illinois School of Professional Psychology (Williams, 2013; Simmons, 2013; Poole, 2013) has shown a strong correlation between Luke's use of metaphact language and his exploration of issues that are felt but not yet clear. This seems particularly significant since a number of studies suggest that the exploration of felt-sense experiences tends to be related to therapeutic success (Hendricks, 2001). My students' research has also found that Luke's process tends to lead to 'problem resolution' in a way that parallels that of more highly functioning clients (Simmons, 2013; Trytten, 2007).

This work on schizophrenic thought disorder has particular significance, since psychologists have tended to advise that therapists avoid connecting with client language that is non-normative. This work suggests that by doing that they may be stopping clients from processing the most significant issues in their lives.

Psychotic self

I have a less clear sense of psychotic self being distinctly different from psychotic process than I do with fragile and dissociated process. Still, I find that my client Luke has a poignant sense of his psychotic self as being distinct from the self before he had a psychotic break in his late teens. He would have trouble saying exactly what is different. But he senses that something overwhelming and tragic happened to him. He once commented that his brothers 'went on to philosophy while he went on to ambulances ...'. When he is feeling emotionally well, he sometimes comments that he feels like the 'old Luke'.

References

Bowlby, J (1969) *Attachment*. New York: Basic Books.

Bowlby, J (1988) Attachment, communication and therapeutic process. In J Bowlby (Ed) *A Secure Base: Clinical applications of attachment theory*. London: Routledge.

Braun, BG (1986) *Treatment of Multiple Personality Disorder*. Washington, DC: American Psychiatric Press.

Coffeng, T (1996) Experiential and pre-experiential therapy for multiple trauma. In R Hutterer, G Pawlowsky, PF Schmid & R Stipsits (Eds) *Client-Centered and Experiential Psychotherapy: A paradigm in motion* (pp. 499–511). Frankfurt am Main: Peter Lang.

Doidge, N (2007) *The Brain that Changes Itself*. New York: Penguin.

Fogel, A (1982) Affect dynamics in early infancy: Affective tolerance. In T Field & A Fogel (Eds) *Emotion and Early Interaction* (pp. 25–56). Hillsdale, NJ: Lawrence Erlbaum Associates.

Hendricks, MN (2001) Focusing-oriented/experiential psychotherapy. In D Cain & J Seeman (Eds) *Humanistic Psychotherapies: Handbook of research and practice* (pp. 221–51). Washington, DC: American Psychological Association.

Kluft, RP (1985) *Childhood Antecedents of Multiple Personality*. Washington, DC: American Psychiatric Press.

Kohut, H (1971) *The Analysis of the Self*. New York: International Universities Press.

Kohut, H (1984) *How Does Analysis Cure?* Chicago: University of Chicago Press.

Lee, R & Martin, JC (1991) *Psychotherapy after Kohut: A textbook of self psychology*. Hillsdale, NJ: The Analytic Press.

Mahler, MS, Pine, F & Bergman, A (1975) *The Psychological Birth of the Human Infant*. New York: Basic Books.

Main, M (1991) Metacognitive knowledge, metacognitive monitoring, and singular (coherent) multiple model of attachment. In CM Parkes, JS Hinde, & D Marris (Eds) *Attachment across the Life Cycle* (pp. 127–59). London: Tavistock/Routledge.

Poole, K (2013) *Schizophrenia and the APES: Discourse of the disorder in a case study and the application of client-centered therapy.* Unpublished Clinical Research Project: Illinois School of Professional Psychology, Argosy University/Chicago.

Prouty, G (1994) *Theoretical Evolutions in Person-Centered/Experiential Psychotherapy: Applications to schizophrenic and retarded psychoses.* Westport, CT: Praeger.

Prouty, G (2001) A new mode of empathy: Empathic contact. In S Haugh & T Merry (Eds) *Rogers' Therapeutic Conditions: Evolution, theory and practice. Vol 2: Empathy* (pp. 155–62). Ross-on-Wye: PCCS Books.

Prouty, G, Van Werde, D & Pörtner, M (2002) *Pre-Therapy: Reaching contact-impaired clients.* Ross-on-Wye: PCCS Books.

Putnam, FW (1989) *Diagnosis and Treatment of Multiple Personality Disorder.* New York: Guilford Press.

Rogers, CR (1951) A theory of personality and behavior (Chapter 11). In *Client-Centered Therapy: Its current practice, implications, and theory* (pp. 481–533). Boston: Houghton Mifflin.

Rogers, CR (1957) The necessary and sufficient conditions of therapeutic personality change. *Journal of Consulting Psychology, 21*(2), 95–103.

Rogers, CR (1959) A theory of therapy, personality and interpersonal relationships, as developed in the client-centered framework. In S Koch (Ed) *Psychology: A study of science. Vol 3: Formulations of the person and the social context* (pp. 184–256). New York: McGraw-Hill.

Roy, B (1991) A client-centered approach to multiple personality and dissociative process. In L Fusek (Ed) *New Directions in Client-Centered Therapy: Practice with difficult client populations* (Monograph Series 1, pp. 18–40). Chicago: Chicago Counseling and Psychotherapy Center.

Schore, AN (2003) *Affect Development and the Repair of the Self.* New York: WW Norton.

Simmons, S (2013) *Schizophrenic Process: Client-centered therapy and development of a felt sense process in a client diagnosed with schizophrenia.* Unpublished Clinical Research Project, Illinois School of Professional Psychology, Argosy University/Chicago.

Sroufe, LA (1996) *Emotional Development: The organization of emotional life in the early years.* New York: Cambridge University Press.

Trytten, JD (2007) *Schizophrenic Client Process: Phase and cognition patterns in a client-centered therapy session.* Unpublished Clinical Research Project, Illinois School of Professional Psychology, Argosy University/Chicago.

Vanaerschot, G (2004) It takes two to tango: On empathy with fragile processes. *Psychotherapy: Theory, Research, Practice, Training, 41*(2), 112–14.

Warner, MS (1997) Does empathy cure? A theoretical consideration of empathy, processing and personal narrative. In A Bohart & LS Greenberg (Eds) *Empathy Reconsidered: New directions in psychotherapy* (pp. 125–40). Washington, DC: American Psychological Association.

Warner, MS (1998) A client-centered approach to therapeutic work with dissociated and fragile process. In LS Greenberg, JC Watson & G Lietaer (Eds) *Handbook of Experiential Psychotherapy* (pp. 368–87). New York: Guilford Press.

Warner, MS (2000) Client-centred therapy at the difficult edge: Work with fragile and dissociated process. In D Mearns & B Thorne (Eds) *Person-Centred Therapy Today: New frontiers in theory and practice* (pp. 144–71). Thousand Oaks, CA: Sage.

Warner, MS (2001) Empathy, relational depth and difficult client process. In S Haugh & T Merry (Eds) *Rogers' Therapeutic Conditions: Evolution, theory and practice. Vol 2: Empathy* (pp. 181–91). Ross-on-Wye: PCCS Books.

Warner, MS (2002a) Psychological contact, meaningful process and human nature. A reformulation of person-centered theory. In G Wyatt & P Sanders (Eds) *Rogers' Therapeutic Conditions: Evolution, theory and practice, Vol 4: Contact and Perception* (pp. 76–95). Ross-on-Wye: PCCS Books.

Warner, MS (2002b) Luke's dilemmas: A client-centered/experiential model of processing with a schizophrenic thought disorder. In JC Watson, RN Goldman, & MS Warner (Eds) *Client-Centered and Experiential Psychotherapy in the 21st Century: Advances in theory, research and practice* (pp. 459–72). Ross-on-Wye: PCCS Books.

Warner, MS (2005) A person-centered view of human nature, wellness, and psychopathology. In S Joseph & R Worsley (Eds) *Person-Centred Psychopathology: A positive psychology of mental health* (pp. 91–109) Ross-on-Wye: PCCS Books.

Warner, MS & Trytten, JD (2008) Metaphact process: A new way of understanding schizophrenic thought disorder. In G Prouty (Ed) *Emerging Developments in Pre-Therapy* (pp. 118–45). Ross-on-Wye: PCCS Books.

Williams, D (2013) *Client Process: An examination of experiencing in a client-centered session with a client diagnosed with schizophrenia.* Unpublished Clinical Research Project: Illinois School of Professional Psychology, Argosy University/Chicago.

11 The relation between intersubjectivity, imitation, mirror neurons, empathy and Pre-Therapy

Hans Peters

In this chapter I will show that there seems to be a link between intersubjectivity, imitation (as a special kind of intersubjectivity), mirror neurons and Pre-Therapy. Regarding mirror neurons I will focus on the work of Gallese (including his articles from 2000, 2001 and 2003a, b) and Iacoboni (2009), because they explicitly describe the relationship between mirror neurons and empathy. Moreover, mirror neurons can be seen as the neurological basis of Pre-Therapy.

The first part of the chapter describes the importance of imitation by parents for the development of the child and concludes that imitation is not as previously thought, a one-way process, but a question of *mutual* influence. As imitation – an innate capacity – takes place in an intersubjective context, the second part of the chapter will outline the concept of intersubjectivity. The capacity for mutual contact is the more important when we realise that the success of pre-therapeutic reflections might be partly due to a connection with this innate capacity for imitation.

The third part of the chapter is dedicated to the question: What might be the neurological basis for the development of intersubjectivity and, as a consequence, the working of Pre-Therapy? The discussion of this question will be elaborated by the presumed working of mirror neurons.

The chapter ends by linking the aforementioned three issues to Pre-Therapy.

The importance of imitation for child development

Stern and his co-workers

From a psychoanalytic orientation Daniel Stern has made a significant contribution to the research on imitation in connection with the early development of intersubjectivity. In his research the notions of attunement (tuning in a broad sense) and affective attunement (a selective form of attunement) played a central role. As I have stated elsewhere, in Stern's view, 'Parents … do not just imitate the behaviours of the child; there must be an empathic attunement … so that parents will react in a congruent way to the behaviours of the child' (Peters, 2005, p. 69). Reacting in a congruent way means that it is not a matter of strict imitation, as Vliegen and Cluckers (2001) stated. Imitation in the sense of intersubjective communication means that the primary caregiver has to pick up the feelings from the child's behaviour, has to imitate that behaviour in a way that enables the child to understand that the response of the caregiver is about the child's original emotional experience and message, not about the caregiver. What is striking is that the relation between mother and child is mainly described as being essentially from the mother to the child, which gives the impression of a one-way communication process. In the 1985 edition of Stern's book, *The Interpersonal World of the Infant* (1985/2000), he almost exclusively described the way the mother reacted to the baby's behaviour, but not the baby's reaction to the mother. In his later work and that of the Boston Process of Change Study Group, especially the study by Tronick (1998), the reciprocity of the relationship received a much stronger and more realistic emphasis. The study group acknowledged that empathy plays an important role within the domain of psychoanalysis, but Tronick also applied more objective research as, for instance, is seen in his work with regard to emotional connectedness and intersubjectivity and the damaging effect on the mental health of the child if there is a failure to achieve this connectedness. In his view the emotional state of the child is implicitly regulated in a dyadic way.

Vliegen and Cluckers

With the help of a concrete observation, Vliegen and Cluckers (2001), also from a psychoanalytic orientation, explain how a mother and her baby come to a reciprocal attunement which gives them both rest.

During the first nine months parents mainly respond by imitating the behaviour of the baby, thereby communicating to the baby that they understand what he is experiencing. They make clear to the child that they understand what is going on inside the child. The particular affective attunement (as opposed to attunement in the broadest sense) follows this first phase. In the first months, the mother imitates the facial expressions, the gestures, and the vocalisations of the child. The mother imitates what the child is doing, but at the same time this is more than a mere imitation, because an exact imitation is not sufficient to come to interpersonal or intersubjective contact. According to the authors, a strict imitation deals with 'overt behaviour' only, which does not refer to what is going on inside the child. With interpersonal communication three processes must take place:

1.   The parent has to be able to read the child's emotion from his or her behaviour, which means the parent must be able to receive the affective message of the baby.

2. The parent has to emit behaviour which is not a strict imitation but which nevertheless corresponds with the child's expressed behaviour. In other words the parent has to express the same emotional quality.

3. The child must be able to understand that the parent's response is connected to the child's own original emotional experiences and messages.

Only in this way can the child experience that in a significant relationship emotion can be shared and understood in a non-verbal or pre-verbal way (Vliegen & Cluckers, 2001, p. 28).

Vliegen and Cluckers point out that several authors identify how the mother responds to the behaviour of the child in the same modality as the emitted behaviours of the child. For example, when the child vocalises, the mother does the same, and when the child makes a facial expression, the same reaction from the mother can be seen, but these reactions are never exactly the same and thus never stereotypical, reiterative sequences.

Client-centred therapists, especially those who are working with pre-therapeutic reflections, will recognise that the three processes mentioned above are also basic processes in the application of Pre-Therapy, although the third process is severely disturbed in most clients who are indicated for Pre-Therapy. In such situations the therapist attempts to connect with the client's remaining contact possibilities. (This will be returned to in the final part of the chapter.)

Gergely and Watson

Gergely and Watson (1996/2004), originally working from a psychoanalytical frame of reference and strongly influenced by learning theory, outline the development of emotional self-awareness and self-control in children. Gergely and Watson find that mutual influence plays an even greater part than previous authors emphasise. The child learns to perceive the affective-emotional expression mirrored by the parent and makes connections with past experiences and anticipated events. However, as the parent usually expresses multiple behaviours simultaneously or nearly simultaneously, the child will develop a detection system that allows him to choose from these different behaviours and, if necessary, link them to what is advantageous to him, what they term the *contingency detection system*. This involves the detection of previously related experiences: '... the baby has shown that only the parent will tend to mirror empathically when the baby is actively expressing a certain negative emotion. For example, the child remembers that anxiously crying always led to empathic reflections on the part of the parents' (Peters, 2003a, p. 90). This remembering should not so much be seen as a conscious act, but more akin to what Damasio describes as the *somatic marker hypothesis*, namely, '... the ability to reason and make decisions in which the (intuitive) feeling is involved' (Peters, 2009, p. 13). The somatic marker draws your attention to possible positive or negative effects of an action. It is primarily an automatic, unconscious, or at most subconscious, alarm signal. It is a system of automatic qualification of predictions, with intuition as a prime example.

In addition, the child is able to anticipate whether his emotional behaviour will result in mirroring behaviour by the parent. Here Gergely and Watson (1996/2004) believe that children, by externalising their internal, emotional states and by experiencing the subsequent reaction of the parents, in due course become able to successfully regulate their emotions, even those that might be perceived as more negative.

But how do the inner, originally unconscious, emotional states in children become conscious? Or, in the words of the authors, '... in what way would the presentation of an external emotional display that is contingent upon the baby's internal affect-state lead to the sensation to and recognition of the internal state that was not consciously accessible before?' (p. 1190). One of these processes is what is called the *biofeedback training procedures*. The originally internal emotional states of the child are exhibited by the child and are subsequently mirrored by the parent. The repeated mirroring by the parent of the same categorical emotional state of the child will lead to the child recognising his or her own feelings, '... and in certain cases subsequent *control over* the internal state' (p. 1190). Gergely and Watson's proposal is '... that parental affect mirroring provides a kind of *natural social feedback training* ... that plays a crucial role in emotional development' (p. 1190). In summary, we can distil the scheme below from Gergely and Watson's text:

> The reviewed findings indicate that during their first year of life infants:
> a. show an innate tendency to express their emotion-states automatically
> b. are sensitive to the contingency structure of face-to-face affective communications
> c. can discriminate discrete facial patterns of emotion expression
> d. are, to a large extent, dependent on their parent's affective-regulative interactions as a means of emotional self-regulation and
> e. the quality of their emerging self-regulative reactions are strongly influenced by the characteristics of their parent's affective communicative behaviour.
>
> (Cited in Peters, 2003a, p. 90)

The detection system, the ability to anticipate and the natural social feedback training can be seen as the basis of the child's ability to manipulate his or her environment, which within certain limits, is positive for his development. By learning that he may have influence on his environment the infant learns to distinguish himself from others. Suppressing the manipulative behaviour in early childhood may be unhelpful as it does not stimulate the child's development. In case the manipulative behaviour is too strong and detrimental to the child and/ or his environment, trying to regulate it may only be necessary as a last resort.

Both Vliegen and Cluckers and Gergely and Watson describe a developmental model which can serve as a framework for understanding why Pre-Therapy is important. Client-centred therapists might do well to be aware of this developmental model and psychoanalytic therapists might also benefit from understanding the value of Pre-Therapy in the treatment of severely contact-disturbed people. There is a considerable amount of literature on this subject, for instance by Peters (1999, 2001), Prouty (1994, 2008) and Prouty, Van Werde and Pörtner, (2002).

From a research point of view

The ideas described so far are mainly written in a one-way direction: the parent imitates the child. However there are many studies (e.g., by Bråten, 1988a, b, 1998a, b; Heimann, 1997, 1998; Kugiumutzakis, 1998; Trevarthen, 1998) showing that even at two hours old, children consciously and unconsciously imitate movements, sounds and the behaviours of parents. Kugiumutzakis describes experimental studies investigating the possibility that imitation could be observed with neonates less than 45 minutes old. The results show that imitative responses, although present in spontaneous neonatal behaviour, occur significantly more often in the presence of the corresponding model than in its absence. This is the case regardless of whether they were born naturally or by caesarean section and whether they were full term or pre-term. From this research children are seen to use two strategies of attention:

1. The majority of the neonates try – with a real observable effort – to direct their attention to the moving part of the experimenter's face. The attention intensifies from a relatively fixed gaze to selective visual exploration. The baby inspects the moving part of the experimenter's face with clear interest while frowning.

2. In the case of facial models, the infant looks at the movement hastily as if it observes only the first presentation, whereupon it immediately starts reproducing the model.

From research, Bråten suggested as early as 1988 that the basic organisation of the mind is both dialogical and intersubjective and that the infant has an innate capacity to take part in an immediate dialogic 'dance' with the other:

> The mother and the infant are seen as one unit of dialogic closure that is organized in a dyadic form already from birth ... which makes it possible to observe proto-conversation already during the first month of life. The infant has the ability to act in a complementary way and the participants step into each other's dialogic circle. (Cited in Heimann, 1998, p. 91 et seq.)

This is important for Pre-Therapy because bringing a dialogical contact into being with severely contact-disturbed clients is the intention of Pre-Therapy.

In line with the research by Bråten, Trevarthen, and others, Heimann conducted research into two questions:

1. Is neonatal imitation in any way directly related to imitation observed during the first year of life?

2. Could we expect children with autism to show an ability to imitate at birth?

The basic assumptions for his research are:

a. that newborn infants are able to imitate facial gestures and that this capacity probably is based on the infant's sensitivity to facial configurations (Johnson & Morton, 1991)

b. the existence of innate social motives (Trevarthen, 1993, 1998), and

c. an innate dialogical organisation of the infant's mind (Bråten, 1988a).

The data of observations from Heimann's research suggest that there are good grounds for accepting neonatal imitation as one example of the infant's innate socio-emotional competence. The data analysis shows that imitation at birth is related to the child's imitative tendency three months later. 'However, we cannot with any certainty state that neonatal imitation has any bearing on the child's psychological development beyond the infancy period' (Heimann, 1998, p. 92). He agrees with Holmlund (1995) who '... submits that imitation is congenital and should be considered as an important part of the early social and communicative interactions taking place between the child and his/her parents' (Holmlund, cited in Heimann, 1998, p. 91). In addition, research shows that neonatal imitation is not a reflexive response, because it is not emitted in the same way in different investigations.

With regard to the second question, Heimann suggests the possibility of two models:

1. The model presented by Bråten '... indicates that the child is born with a dialogical mind which enables him or her to display neonatal imitation, to engage in an immediate dialogical 'dance' and to show primary intersubjectivity' (Heimann, 1998, p. 100). It is not possible to distinguish a child who will later develop autism from a typically developing child during the first weeks or months of life. However, owing to a faulty development of the nervous system some paths of normal brain development are arrested and a deviant route is

taken. According to this scenario a child who develops autism '...
will probably not start to display deviant imitation until he or she is
close to reaching the level of secondary intersubjectivity (somewhere
around 7 to 9 months)' (p. 101).

2. Heimann's second possible path to autism is that the child is born with
    a central nervous system that is already different. The child is not able
    to enter into reciprocal interactions or to display neonatal imitation.
    In this case a lack of imitative responsiveness at birth is a possible
    marker of autism. (Below we will see that Gallese and Iacoboni see a
    possible disorder of mirror neurons being responsible for this.)

Whiten and Brown (1998) conducted research on imitative behaviour in autistic
children compared with normal children and children with mild learning
disabilities. They used the Do-as-I-Do test, developed by Custance, Whiten and
Bard (1994). The first thing that emerges is that a general deficit in imitation in
autism is not supported. On the contrary, autistic children and adults performed
well. Only the young autistic children (under 3 years of age) performed poorly,
but nevertheless about half of their answers produced an attempt to imitate and
some of the answers got the highest score, '... some imitative competence appears
largely intact in all except the young autistic sample' (Whiten & Brown, 1998, p.
270).

Trevarthen built on research from 1969 to 1972 by Bateson (1971, 1975,
1979) in relation to *proto-conversation*. Bateson discovered spontaneous face-to-
face interaction between an infant of 2 to 3 months and the mother, by means of
patterned vocal, facial and gestural expressions. So, it is a way to communicate
before there has been any use of words. In line with earlier studies by Wolff (1963)
and Papousek (1967), Trevarthen describes research from which we learn that
the infant was not producing single reflex responses, nor was smiling or looking
triggered by any identifiable simple sign stimulus:

> Peter Wolff (1963) showed that smiling and 'non-nutritive sucking' were
> reciprocal communicative behaviours from birth. Papousek (1967)
> recorded that when infants were working in an operant procedure, they
> made emotional expressions that communicated their cognitive effort and
> feelings about results 'in a human way'. (Trevarthen, 1998, p. 26)

In 1979 Trevarthen described a 'specifically human system for person-to-
person communication' appearing long before the infant can speak, but with
'rudiments of speech activity' as well. *Pre-speech* – i.e., lip and tongue movements
resembling adult articulation movements and coupled with expressive head
and eye movements and hand gestures – was illustrated with pictures of a girl
7 weeks old. Trevarthen called the expression of individual consciousness and
intentionality *subjectivity* and he concluded that, 'In order to communicate,

infants must also be able to adapt or fit this subjective control to the subjectivity of others: they must also demonstrate *intersubjectivity*' (Trevarthen, 1979, p. 27). According to Trevarthen, Bateson interpreted the infant's behaviour as an innate emotive foundation for language and learning of culture, and for the making of emotionally regulated, and emotional health-regulating, social bonds.

Iacoboni cites an important study by Eckerman and Didow (1996), which shows strong ties between imitation and verbal communication in children. When toddlers who do not know how to speak interact, they tend to play imitation games. 'The more a toddler plays imitation games, the more the same child will be a fluent speaker a year or two later. Imitation seems like the prelude and the facilitator of verbal communication among young children' (Iacoboni, 2009, p. 50).

Intersubjectivity

The Boston Process of Change Study Group, among them Lyons-Ruth and Tronick, gave an ample definition of intersubjectivity. According to Tronick, '... the reader may actually choose their favourite term because there is a vast vagueness associated with many terms – connectedness, intersubjectivity, social contact, attunement, emotional synchrony, reciprocity, attachment – that for the moment need to be dealt with' (Tronick, 1998, p. 292).

In my opinion the meanings of intersubjectivity are most clearly explained in a chapter by Gómez (1998). Working from a developmental psychological framework he defined subjectivity in two different ways.

One-way versus two-way intersubjectivity[1]

Gómez (1998) defined intersubjectivity as the way we perceive, think about, and feel about the world. Someone becomes intersubjective when their subjectivity is capable of taking the subjectivity of others as its object, that is, 'when my mind thinks about the minds of other subjects, or when I feel about the minds or the feelings of others' (Gómez, 1998, p. 245). In this case, it is a question of one-way intersubjectivity. As already acknowledged, Stern's work mainly presents this one-way intersubjectivity. A second expression of intersubjectivity appears when two people are reciprocally aware of each other's awareness – when they are in dialogue – the so-called two-way or second-person intersubjectivity. In other words, '... not all interactions between social agents necessarily entail intersubjectivity' (Meltzoff & Moore, 1998, p. 48). They give the following example: If a baby climbs on the shoulder of its mother, using her simply as a footstool, one cannot speak of intersubjectivity because it is not the other's mind that has been taken into account. Much of the purposeful contact of autistic people is, in consequence,

---

1. The following two sections have been published previously (Peters, 2008).

not intersubjective. As far as I know, Gómez is the first to explicitly make this distinction between one-way and two-way intersubjectivity. Properly speaking, every therapeutic relationship has to develop into two-way intersubjectivity for it to be called a full-fledged relationship.

Cognitive versus affective intersubjectivity

Gómez describes two other aspects of intersubjectivity. First, there is the *theory of mind* (ToM) notion: according to this, some authors think that any appraisal of another's subjectivity must be based on some sort of theoretical knowledge of the other person's mind – as opposed to direct perception or primary representation – whereas others share the idea that knowledge of other minds must be based on some kind of abstract representations, usually referred to as *meta-representations* (Gómez, 1998, pp. 246–7). Both cases deal with theoretical constructs that are not directly observable. This approach of intersubjectivity focuses on the thinking side of people, as perceived by the observer. This is, at least partly, in accordance with Stern's original 1985 notion of intersubjectivity '... beginning around nine months of age with the advent of interattentionality (e.g., pointing), interintentionality (e.g., expecting motives to be read) and interaffectivity (e.g., affect attunement and social referencing)' (Stern, 1985/2000, p. xxii).

The second aspect of intersubjectivity deals with different approaches that focus on *the perception and feeling of emotions*, rather than on the construction of a theory of mind, which, according to Gómez (1998), was the original notion of intersubjectivity. This second notion of intersubjectivity is especially observable in children at a very early stage:

> The subjectivity of others is *felt* by infants, who are capable of attuning themselves to it, in the same way as they display their own subjectivity by means of emotional behaviours to which adults adjust themselves. In Trevarthen's view ... an emotional intersubjectivity precedes and is inseparable from the 'intellectual' intersubjectivity studied by authors working under the label of 'theory of mind'. This emotional intersubjectivity is usually displayed in dialogical situations .... (p. 247)

This overlaps with Stern's later notion of intersubjectivity which stated that new evidence on other-centred participation, as well as the new findings on mirror neurons and adaptive oscillators, convinced him '... that early forms of intersubjectivity exist from almost the beginning of life' (Stern, 1985/2000, p. xxii). This primary intersubjectivity as Stern, in imitation of Trevarthen, called it '... starts from the beginning, as does the sense of an emergent self, as does the sense of a core self ...' (ibid.).

Gómez explicitly distinguishes between emotional and intellectual intersubjectivity and also connects them as being inseparable from each other.

For ToM (theory of mind) theorists, the earliest manifestation of intersubjectivity 'is usually taken to occur at around 9–12 months, when infants start pointing out things to people and engaging in a number of behaviours that are identified under the label of "joint attention"' (Gómez, 1998, p. 248). These theorists underlined the cognitive side of intersubjectivity. Advocates of the emotional approaches of intersubjectivity (the *primary* intersubjectivity, already extant before three or four months) emphasise the expressive and affective components, that is they not only speak in terms of reaching, pointing, or looking to the face 'but also in terms of complying with instructions, accepting assistance, acquiescing, resisting, or making facial expressions' (ibid., p. 249). In this view, one can certainly speak of awareness and of symbolisation, which could, of course, be pre-verbal. Below we will see that it is also the start of empathy.

Intersubjectivity and mirror neurons

The previous section outlines views partly confirmed by research as well as others which presently remain still largely hypotheses. Rizzolatti, Gallese and Iacoboni have all made large neurological contributions regarding intersubjectivity working in the field of *mirror neurons*. Imitative learning, seen as a form of intersubjectivity, '... requires learning a novel movement for your motor repertoire by watching somebody else performing the movement' according to Iacoboni (2009, p. 39). According to Ferrari, Gallese, Rizzolatti and Fogassi (2003), mirror neurons appear to play a crucial role.

A possible neurological basis for intersubjectivity

In 1998 Heimann wrote that the neurological foundation of imitation is '... a direct process at a subcortical level where visual, auditory and somatosensory information share the same neural maps or even the same multimodal neurons' (p. 103). Heimann's statement seems to fit with the discovery of *mirror neurons* by an Italian research group under the direction of Vittorio Gallese. In the early 1990s Gallese et al., investigating hand movements in monkeys, discovered by chance that neurons in the brains of a monkey were active even if the monkey did not move. It turned out that the monkey had observed one of the co-workers and that neural activities were executed *as if* the monkey himself executed the observed movements of the person. Further investigation revealed that such processes also took place in the human brain. In other words, when we observe a person's activities, then, on a neural level, we mirror the observed actions exhibited by the other.

> ... that agency plays an important role in establishing meaningful bonds among individuals, by enabling them with a direct, automatic, non-predicative, and non-inferential simulation mechanism, by means of which the observer can recognize and understand the behaviours of others. (Gallese, 2000, p. 12)

Originally it was thought that this process happens only if the observed action is goal-related behaviour. For instance, observing grasping at a cup in order to get hold of it has to be seen as a goal-oriented action, otherwise such neural process will not take place in the observer: '... these neurons do not respond to static presentations of hand or objects, but require, in order to be triggered, the observation of meaningful, goal-related hand–object interactions' (Gallese, 2000, p. 2). This was confirmed when such behaviour was executed by a mechanical agent or a tool: in these cases mirror neurons were not activated. According to Gallese, this means it is the goal-oriented motor activity, not the visual perception of the object, which is decisive for activating these mirror neurons. In other words, if the goal orientation of the motor activity is not subconsciously recognised by the observer, no mirror neurons will be activated: '... the observed action cannot be matched on the observer's motor repertoire, and therefore the intended goal cannot be detected and/or attributed to the mechanical agent' (2000, p. 3). The latter is partly refuted by Gilbert amongst others. He demonstrated that the use of tools gave the same results *when the observer can perceive the goal-oriented nature of the action*. 'This is facilitated by incorporation of the tool in the body scheme. Body scheme is the way in which the neural control (the brain) configures the body' according to Gilbert (2004, p. 63). Ferrari et al. (2003) also discovered that about 20 per cent of the mirror neurons do also respond when the actions are executed by a tool. However extensive experiments by Bekkering and his colleagues (Bekkering, Wohlschläger & Gattis, 2000; Wohlschläger & Bekkering, 2002; Koski, et al., 2002) and Iacoboni (2009) demonstrate that goal-oriented processes prevail.

Gallese pointed out, following Perret et al. (1989), that the part of the brain that has long been considered exclusively for motor action also appears to have detection capabilities through mirror neurons. In addition, Broca's area is not only involved in language mastery, but also in analysing people's pre-linguistic behaviour. Research by both Meltzoff (1995) and Gallese shows that this capacity already exists in 18-month-old children.

Further investigation by Gallese also revealed that such imitation processes seem not limited to grasping, but that many other physical and mental states involved in our relating to others, such as emotions, body schema, the experience of pain and other somatic sensations, are shared (or might be shared, H.P.) situations. Gallese's thesis is that the many aspects through which we can identify our self with others have one common root, namely *empathy*.

Thus, fundamental functional qualities of most neurons in certain areas of the brain do not discharge in direct relation to primary feelings, but rather to the observation of goal-oriented behaviours. This implicit process of pre-reflexive, simulated action is of great interest for the development of behaviour from birth onwards (for instance, with regard to imitation), for the recognition of behaviour of one's own species (social identity) and for the development of one's own identity. In short, for the development of intersubjectivity this implicit process is a very important one. Gallese pointed out that research findings revealed that not only are motor neurons involved, but also that audio-visual mirror neurons act in the same way. They laid the neurobiological foundation to identify oneself with the other while maintaining one's own identity (i.e., empathy).

Empathy and mirror neurons

As early as 1903, Lips wrote that empathy was characterised by an inner imitation of movements observed in others. Gallese indicates that this is not restricted to motor acts and that the neural mirror system not only holds for motor acts, but that '... sensations and emotions displayed by others can also be "empathized" with, and therefore *implicitly* understood through a mirror matching mechanism' (Gallese, 2003a, p. 176). This mechanism, which he sees as a driving force in the cognitive and psychological development of more sophisticated forms of intersubjective relationships that lead to social identity, led him to extend the concept of empathy '... in order to accommodate and account for *all* different aspects of expressive behaviour enabling us to establish a meaningful link between others and ourselves' (p. 176 et seq.). In other words, our reactions to experiences that we obtain in dealing with others and that are affecting our own thinking, feeling, acting and reacting to others, are prepared on a neural level, even before we are aware of them.

Whether this so-called 'extension of the concept of empathy' is really an enlargement of the notion of empathy or whether the view that Gallese stands for has always been implicitly captured in this concept is debatable. Either way, neither in Rogers' first descriptions of empathy nor in any subsequent description by other authors is the origin of empathy explained. De Waal described empathy as an evolutionary developed ability coming into being far before man in his current capacity arose or 'Empathy is part of our evolution ... an age-old innate ability. Relying on an automatic sensitivity to faces, bodies and voices, people have known empathy from the very beginning' (de Waal, 2010, p. 227). To experience empathy, it is necessary for the other to manifest themselves in some way, however subtle, in behaviours or emotional expressions, before we will be able to empathise with him or her. The basis for this is, according to Iacoboni, the intimacy of imitation: 'The intimacy of self and other that imitation and mirror neurons facilitate may be the first step toward empathy' (Iacoboni, 2009, p. 70). Iacoboni also states that the study of early human development '... shows how powerfully imitation is connected with the development of important social skills. ... If imitation is so critical to develop these social skills, mirror neurons that enable imitation must be too', according to Iacoboni (ibid.). During the neural activity of mirror neurons, signals are sent to the emotional areas in the limbic system which enable us to feel and recognise emotions, (e.g., the perception of a smile is associated with happiness, and a frown with sadness).

'Only *after* we feel these emotions internally are we able to explicitly recognize them' (Iacoboni, 2009, p. 112, my italics).

Gallese and Iacoboni describe how inside, on a neural level, a process takes place that matches with the activities and experiences of the person observed by us, in such a way that we are able to understand the other as if we are him/her. De Waal even speaks of identification as a porch for empathy: 'Identification with others opens the door to empathy, the absence of identification slams that door shut' (2010, p. 95, my translation). Those imitated interactions and the identification with the other do not in any way imply merging with each other. Iacoboni sees the role that mirror neurons play in providing the possibility of intersubjectivity as interdependence. This is, at least partly, in line with Heyes' idea and research on the development of mirror neurons, namely that the mirror neuron system is a product, as well as a process, of social interaction, known as the *associative hypothesis* (Heyes, 2010).

It is important to be aware that it remains unclear exactly how this works. Gradually more publications are emerging from researchers who, despite their proven sympathy to the theory of mirror neurons, make critical investigations into *how* they work. This group includes, among others, Berthouze, Borenstein and Ruppin, 2005 (evolutionary link between mirror neurons and imitation); the aforementioned Gilbert, 2004 (the cognitive dimension of consciousness and mirror neural effects) and Heyes, 2010 (see above).

Shared manifold hypothesis of intersubjectivity

From the above-mentioned ideas Gallese developed his *shared manifold hypothesis of intersubjectivity* (SMH) (Gallese, 2000, 2001, 2003a, b). In short, this means that when we enter into a mutual relationship, we share a multiplicity of states which Gallese defines as 'implicit certainties'. 'We share emotions, our body schema, our being subject to somatic sensations such as pain. ... It is just because of this shared manifold that intersubjective communication, social imitation and ascription of intentionality become possible' (Gallese, 2003a, p. 177). This implies, as we saw previously, that the operation of the neural mechanisms involved in the interaction with others not only plays a role in motor activities, but also in the audio-visual field and other sensory sensations. One of the levels that the shared manifold can be operationalised on is the phenomenological or empathic level: 'Actions, emotions and sensations experienced by others become implicitly meaningful to us because we can share them with others' (ibid.). This is in line with the view that the functioning of the neural mechanisms that play a role in the interaction with others is not only based on motor, but also on audio-visual and tactile areas (see, among others, Gazzola, Aziz-Zadeh & Keysers, 2006). Iacoboni (2009) speaks of *stimulus enhancement*: the content of what is displayed is independent of the ways in which the content emerges; in other words, independent of the plurality of modes of expression. He gives the example of mirror neurons that not only fire if the animal sees the breaking of a peanut, but also when they only hear the breaking sound. This means a significant extension of the neural level of mutual understanding and experiencing or, as Gallese states, 'sameness of content is shared with different organisms ... mirror neurons instantiate a multimodel representation of organism–organism relations' (2003a, p. 175). This takes place in a common intersubjective space that he refers to as *we-centric*. Although developmental psychology has shown that the agreement between the self and the other (the self–other analogy) is heavily reliant on action and imitation of action, it is not restricted to the domain of action. Global physical sensations and a multitude of affects described as a '... broad range of "implicit certainties" we entertain about other individuals, all contributing to compose our global shared experiential dimension with others' (ibid.). Gallese calls this multi-dimensional aspect of self–other relationships *the shared manifold of intersubjectivity* and quotes Depraz who states that '... the self-other identity at the level of the body enables an intersubjective transfer of meaning to occur. From the very onset of life, subjectivity is intersubjectivity' (ibid.).

Psychopathological implications

Researchers have been interested in whether there are any implications for the aetiology of different presentations. For example, whether the person who presents as sociopathic and is displaying little or no empathy for the environment has a different brain structure, a dysfunction of the neural system or whether this representation is entirely determined by the environment. It is known from the work of Damasio (2004a, b) amongst others that damage to certain brain areas can lead to severe emotional disturbances and the absence of empathic feeling. In particular, disorders in the amygdala can lead to a lack of empathic ability.

Iacoboni reports how the neurophysiological properties of mirror neurons in monkeys observed by a Scottish group of experts, the observed imitation shortages in autistic children and the brain imaging experiments on imitation led them to hypothesise '... an early developmental failure of the mirror neuron system that would subsequently result in a cascade of developmental impairments leading to autism' (2009, p. 173). People on the autism spectrum are also unable to make a translation to the perspective of the other, nor do they tend to look to their caretakers or link their own movements with the movements of people that imitate them. As reported earlier, Whiten and Brown (1998) showed that children with an autism spectrum disorder are in principle able to imitate, and Iacoboni (2009) considers certain forms of treatment based on imitation effective.

Gallese identifies a clear lack of experienced 'unity in diversity' of self and the other in people diagnosed with schizophrenia (Gallese, 2003a, p. 177) and like Stanghellini (2000) views schizophrenia as involving problems with *attunement*:

> ... the incapacity to engage oneself in meaningful relations with others, the impossibility to establish precognitive, non-inferential, 'intuitive' interpersonal bonds. ... by emphasizing the *relational character* of the psychopathology of schizophrenia, this approach has the merit to disclose the possibility to establish a more insightful therapeutic bond with psychotic patients. (Gallese, 2003a, p. 178)

A possible cause is a disruption of the multilevel simulation processes that characterise the shared manifold. 'If the mechanisms enabling us to constitute the implicit certainties we normally entertain about the world do not function properly, we are left with a need to *purposively* attribute a sense to a world that looks totally strange' (ibid.).

Client-centred therapy and in particular Pre-Therapy can make a meaningful contribution to responding to these issues (see for instance, Peters, 2001, 2003b, 2008; Prouty, Van Werde & Pörtner, 1998, 2002; Prouty, 1994, 2008).

The innate capacity for intersubjective imitation in relation to Pre-Therapy

Introduction

Pre-Therapy, as a form of client-centred/experiential psychotherapy, is applied to clients with severe innate or acquired contact disturbances, for whom the more conventional forms of therapy such as talking therapy and behaviour therapy are not (yet) applicable. The almost complete absence of contact (Prouty, 1994, 2008, called this *existential autism*) makes the application of these kinds of treatment impossible. So the therapist first has to establish or restore the client's very basic contact functions, what can be described as the *primary application* of Pre-Therapy (Peters, 1999). Because some form of contact is a precondition (therefore the use of the prefix 'pre' in Pre-Therapy) for the more conventional forms of therapy, the question is how to bring this contact into being with clients who are severely disturbed, have hallucinatory psychoses or who have learning disabilities with contact disturbances, and so on. Such contact is the goal of pre-therapeutic work. This is done by the application of pre-therapeutic reflections, the so-called *contact reflections* (for an extended description of the contact reflections see, among others, Peters, 1999, 2008; Prouty, 1994, 2008 and this volume). From his or her own congruence, the therapist mirrors the minimal behavioural utterances of the client, expressions he or she also bodily 'radiates' but which are not bodily experienced. If a certain level of contact is possible, especially word-for-word and facial reflections can play an important role in the current, individual verbal therapies, for example, in clients with short consciousness decreases, the so-called secondary application of Pre-Therapy.

Intersubjectivity, imitation and Pre-Therapy

So Pre-Therapy is a kind of client-centred/experiential psychotherapy aiming at restoring or bringing about primary or secondary contact in an intersubjective context. The relation between intersubjectivity and Pre-Therapy is well illustrated by this quote from Prouty:

> Pre-Therapy ... can be understood in the following way:
>> Pre-Therapy is a form of attunement on very young levels of development
>> Pre-Therapy is a form of intersubjective contact
>> Pre-Therapy is an intersubjective relationship
>> Mirror neurons are the empathic basis for Pre-Therapy
> (Prouty, 2008, p. 86)

Pre-Therapy is mainly applicable to people with (severe) contact disturbances – that is, a nearly total lack of contact with themselves and with the surrounding world. A large part of the target group consists of people with learning disabilities and/or people with an autistic contact disturbance. This means that the therapist often takes the initiative to have contact with the client, which is a kind of one-way intersubjectivity, hoping that this will lead to two-way intersubjectivity. With people suffering from a severe contact crisis, especially with people who are mentally handicapped, the cognitive disturbance is predominantly present. This means that the second form of intersubjectivity, which focuses on the perception and feeling of emotions, is the central topic in this kind of treatment rather than the cognitive form of intersubjectivity. This second form of intersubjectivity already exists in the neonate.

We have seen that both imitation and the development of intersubjectivity belong to people's neonatal capacities, including those with learning disabilities and/or autism. This means that the therapist, in applying pre-therapeutic contact reflections, can both join with the remaining behaviours the client exhibits, and appeal to the innate skills that people have at their disposal: imitation and intersubjectivity are archaic potentialities that humans possess. These capacities develop relatively spontaneously in the neonate, whereas in a person with severe contact disturbances these capacities are blocked and have to be evoked. Imitation of the limited utterances of the neonate by the mother (which supports the development of mutual intersubjectivity) corresponds with the application of pre-therapeutic reflections by the therapist. Both an attuned caregiver and a pre-therapist link into behaviours that are close to the person and that might elicit a response. This can be seen as the foundation of the success of pre-therapeutic interventions.

An obvious question is whether pre-therapeutic reflections rest too much on a mechanical imitation of the client's behaviour. One can ask the same question concerning the imitative behaviour of the mother. We have already seen that the imitation by the mother is not a strict imitation of the child's behaviour, but her imitation is coloured by her empathic feeling and by her congruent way of responding. This is analogous to the application of pre-therapeutic reflections. The therapist approaches the client in an empathic and accepting way, joins with the basal rest behaviours the client exhibits; however, at the same time, the therapist approaches the client from his or her own congruence so that therapist and client do not coincide. It is what Rogers (1962) and Kohut (1977) called *mirroring*.

With reference to infants, Gergely and Watson (1996) thought that there is evidence that infants are extremely sensitive to the difference between their own affective–expressive utterances and those of the parents. As we have seen, this is in line with Vliegen and Cluckers' view. At a very early stage, the child seems able to see the responses of the mother as corresponding with his or her own feelings and behaviours, but also as differing from them. This has a direct parallel with the application of pre-therapeutic reflections. The therapist links up with the behaviours of the client but in doing so also acts in empathic orientation to the client and from his or her own congruence. This gives the client the best opportunity to recognise the behaviours of the therapist as part of the client, him or herself, which will facilitate client responsiveness. On the other hand, the client also has to distinguish his or her affective-emotional utterances from those of the therapist. This is essential because the client has to learn that the reality contact is his or her reality within the context of his or her existence and not the therapist's.

Summarising conclusions

My tentative conclusions are the following:

- As seen in the aforementioned work of authors such as Bråten, Trevarthen, Kugiumutzakis, Heimann, Meltzoff and Moore, and others, there is sufficient proof that imitation and intersubjectivity are innate human capacities.

- These capacities are accessible from the very first hours of life.

- These basic capacities also exist in people who are autistic and/or those having learning disabilities. (The strong tendency by children with Down's syndrome to imitate is especially well known.)

- With these clients, as well as with the clients who are severely contact disturbed, the emotional view of intersubjectivity is far more important than the intellectual one. In other words, approaches where the perception and feeling of emotions are central (which is, according to Gómez, 1998, the original conception of intersubjectivity) are situated on an earlier developmental level in which pre-speech and proto-conversation play a relatively important role.

- The neonate has the capacity to distinguish the caregiver's responses as differing from as well as corresponding to their own behaviours.

- Research has shown that imitation can be seen as a mutually influencing and dialogical process, and this connects well with the concept of Pre-Therapy. The intention of Pre-Therapy is to bring about a contact dialogue, after which the more regular forms of psychotherapy may be applicable.

- Pre-therapeutic reflections are therefore in line with the very basic imitative and intersubjective capacities which exist in human beings from birth.

- The caregiver's imitation of a child's vocalising is attuned and not a pure mechanical repetition of these behaviours. Similarly, in Pre-Therapy, the therapist reflects the often minimal behaviours of the client from an empathic stance and in their own congruent way.

- Further research into the way mirror neurons work would make an important contribution to the understanding of the functioning of imitation and the success of Pre-Therapy.

So, Pre-Therapy can be seen from a developmental frame of reference in which the success of the application of pre-therapeutic reflections, even with adults, proceeds because they are attuned to the basic potentialities we have from birth.

References

Bateson, MC (1971) The interpersonal context of infant vocalization. *Quarterly Progress Report of the Research Laboratory of Electronics, 100,* 170–6.

Bateson, MC (1975) Mother–infant exchanges: The epigenesis of conversational interaction. In D Aaronson & RW Rieber (Eds) *Developmental Psycholinguistics and Communication Disorders* Vol. 153 (pp. 101–13). New York: Academy of Sciences.

Bateson, MC (1979) 'The epigenesis of conversational interaction': A personal account of research development. In M Bullowa (Ed) *Before Speech* (pp. 63–77). Cambridge: Cambridge University Press.

Bekkering, H, Wohlschläger, A & Gattis, M (2000) Imitation of gestures in children is goal-directed. *The Quarterly Journal of Experimental Psychology, Section A, 53,* 153–64.

Berthouze, L, Borenstein, L & Ruppin, E (2005) The evolution of imitation and mirror neurons in adaptive agents. *Cognitive Systems Research, 6,* 229–42.

Bråten, S (1988a) Dialogic mind: The infant and the adult in protoconversation. In M Carvallo (Ed) *Nature, Cognition and System,* Vol. 1 (pp. 187–205). Dordrecht: Kluwer Academic Publishers.

Bråten, S (1988b) Between dialogic mind and monologic reason: Postulating the virtual Other. In M Campanella (Ed) *Between Rationality and Cognition* (pp. 205–35). Torino: Meynier.

Bråten, S (Ed) (1998a) *Intersubjective Communication and Emotion in Early Ontogeny.* Cambridge: Cambridge University Press.

Bråten, S (1998b) Infant learning by altercentric participation: The reverse of egocentric observations in autism. In S Bråten (Ed) *Intersubjective Communication and Emotion in Early Ontogeny* (pp. 105–27). Cambridge: Cambridge University Press.

Custance, DM, Whiten, A & Bard, KA (1994) The development of gestural imitation and self-recognition in chimpanzees and young children. In JJ Roeder et al (Eds) *Current Primatology,* Vol. II (pp. 381–7). Strasbourg: Université Louis Pasteur.

Damasio, A (2004a) *De Vergissing van Descartes. Gevoel, verstand en het menselijk brein.* Amsterdam: Wereldbibliotheek. (Original work published 1994 in English, *Descartes' Error – Emotion, reason and the human brain.* New York: Putnam's Sons)

Damasio, A (2004b) *Looking for Spinoza. Joy, sorrow and the feeling brain.* London: Vintage.

De Waal, F (2010) *Een Tijd voor Empathie.* Amsterdam/Antwerpen: Uitgeverij Contact.

Eckerman, CO & Didow, SM (1996) 'Nonverbal imitation in toddlers.' Mastery of verbal means of achieving coordinated actions. *Developmental Psychology, 32,* 141–52.

Ferrari, PF, Gallese, G, Rizolatti, G & Fogassi, L (2003) Mirror neurons responding to the observation of ingestive and communicative mouth actions in the monkey ventral premotor cortex. *European Journal of Neuroscience, 17,* 1703–14.

Gallese V (2000) Action, goals, and their role in intersubjectivity: From mirror neurons to the 'shared manifold' hypothesis. Retrieved 23 October 2004 from http://www.mpipf-muenchen.mpg.de/MPIPF/MECA/docs/gallese.doc

Gallese, V (2001) The 'shared manifold' hypothesis. From mirror neurons to empathy. *Journal of Conscious Studies, 8,* 33–50.

Gallese, V (2003a) The roots of empathy: The shared manifold hypothesis and the neural basis of intersubjectivity. *Psychopathology, 36,* 171–80.

Gallese, V (2003b) The manifold nature of interpersonal relations: The quest for a common mechanism. *Phil. Trans. Royal Society London, 358,* 517–28.

Gazzola, V, Aziz-Zadeh, L & Keysers, C (2006) Empathy and the somatotopic auditory mirror system in humans. *Current Biology, 16,* 1824–9.

Gergely, G & Watson, JS (1996) The social biofeedback theory of parental affect mirroring. The development of self-awareness and self-control in infancy. *International Journal of Psychoanalysis, 77,* 1181–212. Also published in Fonagy, P, Gergely, G, Jursit, EL & Target, M (2004) *Affect Regulation, Mentalization, and the Development of the Self.* London/New York: Karnak.

Gilbert, J (2004) *De Cognitieve Dimensie van Bewustzijn en Spiegelneurale Effecten.* Unpublished dissertation. Gent.

Gómez, JC (1998) Do concepts of intersubjectivity apply to non-human primates? In S Bråten (Ed) *Intersubjective Communication and Emotion in Early Ontogeny* (pp. 245–60). Cambridge: Cambridge University Press.

Heimann, M (1997) *The Never Ending Story of Neonatal Imitation.* Poster presented at the VIIIth European Conference on Developmental Psychology. Rennes, France.

Heimann, M (1998) Imitation in neonates, in older infants and in children with autism: Feedback to theory. In S Bråten (Ed) *Intersubjective Communication and Emotion in Early Ontogeny* (pp. 89–105). Cambridge: Cambridge University Press.

Heyes, C (2010) Where do mirror neurons come from? *Neuroscience and Biobehavioral Reviews, 34*(4), 575–83. Retrieved 19th March 2014 from www.sciencedirect.com/science/article/pii/S0149763409001730

Holmlund, C (1995) Development of turntakings as a sensorimotor process in the first 3 months: A sequential analysis. In KE Nelson & Z Réger (Eds) *Children's Language*, Vol. VIII (pp. 41–64). Hillsdale, NY: Earlbaum.

Iacoboni, M (2009) *Mirroring People. The science of empathy and how we connect with others.* New York: Picador. In Dutch (2008) *Het Spiegelende Brein. Overlevingsvermogen, imitatiegedrag en Spiegelneuronen.* Amsterdam: Uitgeverij Nieuwerzijds.

Johnson, MH & Morton, J (1991) *Biology and Cognitive Development.* Oxford: Basil Blackwell.

Koski, L, Wohlschläger, A, Bekkering, H, Woods, RP, Dubeau, MC, Mazziota, JC & Iacoboni, M (2002) Modulation of motor and premotor activity during imitation of target-directed actions. *Cerebral Cortex, 12,* 847–55.

Kohut, H (1977) *The Restoration of the Self.* New York: International University Press.

Kugiumutzakis, G (1998) Neonatal imitation in the intersubjective companion space. In S Bråten (Ed) *Intersubjective Communication and Emotion in Early Ontogeny* (pp. 63–89). Cambridge: Cambridge University Press.

Lips, T (1903) *Grundlegung der Aestetik: 1.* Leipzig: Voss.

Meltzoff, AN (1995) Understanding the intentions of others: Re-enactment of intended acts by 18-month-old children. *Developmental Psychology, 31,* 838–50.

Meltzoff, AN & Moore, MK (1998) Infant intersubjectivity: Broadening the dialogue to include imitation, identity and intention. In S Bråten (Ed) *Intersubjective Communication and Emotion in Early Ontogeny* (pp. 47–63). Cambridge: Cambridge University Press.

Papousek, H (1967) Experimental studies of apparitional behavior in human newborns and infants. In HW Stevenson, EH Hess & HL Rheingold (Eds) *Early Behavior* (pp. 249–77). New York: Wiley & Sons.

Perret, DI, Harries, MH, Bevan, R, Thomas, S, Benson, PJ, Mistlin, AJ, Chitty, AJ, Hietanen, JK & Ortega, JE (1989) Framework of analysis for the neural representation of animate objects and actions. *Journal of Experiential Biology, 146,* 87–113.

Peters, H (1999) Pretherapy: A client-centered/experiential approach to mentally handicapped people. *Journal of Humanistic Psychology, 39,* 8–29.

Peters, H (2001) *Psychotherapeutische Zugänge zu Menschen mit Geistiger Behinderung.* Stuttgart: Klett-Cotta.

Peters, H (2003a) Enkele gedachten over vroegkinderlijk imiteren en intersubjectiviteit in relatie tot aspecten van psychotherapie. *Tijdschrift Cliëntgerichte Psychotherapie, 41,* 84–115.

Peters, H (2003b) Imitatie, intersubjectiviteit en pretherapeutische reflecties: een Samenhang in verschillen. *Tijdschrift Cliëntgerichte Psychotherapie, 41,* 168–80.

Peters, H (2005) Pre-Therapy from a developmental perspective. *Journal of Humanistic Psychology, 45,* 62–81.

Peters, H (2008) The development of intersubjectivity in relation to psychotherapy and its importance for Pre-Therapy. In G Prouty (Ed) *Emerging Developments in Pre-Therapy* (pp. 87–104). Ross-on-Wye: PCCS Books.

Peters, H, (2009) Emoties en gevoelens volgens Damasio: een poging tot samenvatting. *Tijdschrift Cliëntgerichte Psychotherapie, 47,* 5–23.

Prouty, G (1994) *Theoretical Evolutions in Person-Centered/Experiential Therapy. Applications to schizophrenic and retarded psychoses.* New York: Praeger.

Prouty, G (Ed) (2008) *Emerging Developments in Pre-Therapy: A Pre-Therapy reader.* Ross-on-Wye: PCCS Books.

Prouty, G, Van Werde, D & Pörtner, M (1998) *Prä-Therapie.* Stuttgart: Klett-Cotta.

Prouty, G, Van Werde, D & Pörtner, M (2002) *Pre-Therapy: Reaching contact-impaired clients.* Ross-on-Wye: PCCS Books.

Rogers, CR (1962) The interpersonal relationship: The core of guidance. *Harvard Education Review, 3,* 426–41.

Stanghellini, G (2000) Vulnerability to schizophrenia and lack of common sense. *Schizophrenia Bulletin, 26,* 775–87.

Stern, DN (2000) *The Interpersonal World of the Infant: A view from psychoanalysis and developmental psychology* (2nd ed with new introduction). New York: Basic Books. (Original work published 1985)

Trevarthen, C (1979) Communication and cooperation in early infancy: A description of primary intersubjectivity. In M Bullowa (Ed) *Before Speech* (pp. 321–47). London: Academic Press.

Trevarthen, C (1993) The function of emotions in early communication and development. In J Nadel & L Camaioni (Eds) *New Perspectives in Early Communicative Development* (pp. 48–81). London: Routledge.

Trevarthen, C (1998) The concept of foundations of infant intersubjectivity. In S Bråten (Ed) *Intersubjective Communication and Emotion in Early Ontogeny* (pp. 15–47). Cambridge: Cambridge University Press.

Tronick, EZ (1998) Dyadically expanded states of consciousness and the process of therapeutic change. *Infant Mental Health Journal, 19,* 290–300.

Vliegen, N & Cluckers, G (2001) Babyobservatie en therapeutisch proces. Van een historisch perspectief naar een actueel verband. In N Vliegen & C Leroy (Eds) *Het Moederland? De vroegste relatie tussen moeder en kind in de psychoanalytische therapie* (pp. 21–45). Leuven/Leusden: Acco.

Whiten, A & Brown, J (1998) Imitation and the reading of minds: Perspectives from the study of autism, normal children and non-human primates. In S Bråten (Ed) *Intersubjective Communication and Emotion in Early Ontogeny* (pp. 260–80). Cambridge: Cambridge University Press.

Wohlschläger, A & Bekkering, H (2002) Is human imitation based on a mirror-neuron system? Some behavioural evidence. *Experimental Brain Research, 143,* 335–41.

Wolff, PH (1963) Observations on the early development of smiling. In BM Foss (Ed) *The Determinants of Infant Behavior,* Vol 2 (pp. 113–38). London: Methuen.

Refutation of myths of inappropriateness of person-centred therapy at the difficult edge 12

Lisbeth Sommerbeck

Person-centred practitioners will all have heard the statement that, 'person-centred therapy is only for "the worried well"', but not appropriate with more serious problems, that is, with precisely the clients with whom person-centred practitioners often find themselves at a difficult edge. It can therefore be supportive and helpful for these practitioners to know about the arguments that can refute this statement and reveal it for what it is: a myth.

In this chapter I highlight and correct four mistakes made by those who claim that person-centred therapy is only for 'the worried well':

1. the idea that empathic understanding of psychosis colludes with it or reinforces it
2. the confusion of 'non-directive' with 'unstructured'
3. the notion that person-centred therapy is too in-depth and exploratory
4. the confusion of the theory of therapy with the theory of personality.

I will deal with each of these mistakes in turn and in the final section I will give my reasons, from almost 40 years of experience with psychotherapeutic work in a psychiatric hospital, for regarding person-centred therapy as being not only useful with clients diagnosed with serious psychiatric disturbances, but also for regarding person-centred therapy with its pre-therapeutic extension (Prouty, 1994; Prouty, Van Werde & Pörtner, 2002; Sanders, 2007) as the only psychotherapeutic approach that is viable at times with people whom other approaches regard as being 'beyond psychotherapeutic reach'.

This chapter is an adapted version of Sommerbeck, L (2005) An evaluation of research, concepts and experiences pertaining to the universality of CCT and its application in psychiatric settings. In S Joseph & R Worsley (Eds) *Person-Centred Psychopathology* (pp. 317–36). Ross-on-Wye: PCCS Books.

The erroneous notion that empathy colludes with or reinforces psychotic ideation

With the intent of accompanying the client on his or her explorative and developmental journey, the person-centred therapist suspends his or her own conception of reality, putting it in parenthesis in order not to disturb the client's own process. There is, thus, no room for responding from the therapist's own conception of reality, however unfamiliar or mistaken the client's conception of reality may seem to the therapist. This is also the case with clients who present with so-called psychotic ideation, that is, hallucinations and delusions, which do seem extremely unfamiliar to the therapist and quite at odds with the therapist's and others' more-or-less consensual conception of reality. With these clients the therapist's capacity to suspend his or her own conception of reality is put to the test and with these clients it is particularly important to remember that empathic understanding is neutral as far as confirmation or disconfirmation of the client's conception of reality is concerned. Empathic understanding of a client's conception of reality is *not* agreeing with it. Whether the therapist agrees or not is, in person-centred therapy, therapeutically irrelevant. However, I've often seen empathic understanding confused with confirmation, even in psychotherapeutically well-informed circles. For example, the leader of the Danish Psychoanalytic Institute writes that 'empathic confirmation' is useful to strengthen the therapeutic alliance (Vitger, 1999, p. 200).

With a notion of empathic understanding as confirmative it is little wonder that empathic understanding is dismissed as useless and even harmful with clients who present with psychotic ideation. In psychiatric circles there seems to be a widespread fear that you are colluding with or reinforcing psychotic ideation if you respond with expressions of empathic understanding. Instead of expressing empathic understanding, 'reality correction' is the favoured approach, particularly among psychiatric nurses, to patients' expression of psychotic ideation. They often relate to patients as if not doing reality correction is synonymous with collusion with the patients' conceptions of reality.

For people who regard reality correction as a necessary element in the treatment of people diagnosed with psychosis, client-centred therapy is of course seen as inconsequential, at best, and harmful, at worst.

There is, naturally, no guarantee that a client does not experience a therapist's expression of empathic understanding as confirmative (or disconfirmative, for that matter) of the client's conception of reality. It is, though, contrary to the essence of person-centred therapy to try to control client experiences in any way, including client experiences of the therapist. Client experiences of the therapist are received and followed with empathic understanding just like all other client experiences.

Contrary to this myth of collusion, it has been my experience, from my work in a psychiatric hospital, that it is reality correction that is potentially harmful to clients diagnosed with psychosis, not expressions of empathic understanding – and that it is expressions of empathic understanding that are beneficial, not reality correction. Reality correction is, by its very nature, confrontative and patients with a diagnosis of psychosis feel, in general, threatened by confrontative approaches. Faced with reality correction they often tend to defend their conception of reality, thereby rigidifying and solidifying it and often expanding on it with more details and nuances, thereby developing their psychotic ideation further. In short, they can become more psychotic when confronted with reality correction.

In contrast, expression of accurate empathic understanding, non-confrontative as it is, gives the client no reason to defend his or her perception of reality. This is precisely what makes it possible for the client to consider alternative points of view. The client feels that his or her perception of reality is understood and accepted, which leaves the client feeling free to explore it further. In this climate of safety and acceptance, the client will then most often, very tentatively and in very minor ways at first, start to question some inconsistencies that the client discovers in his or her psychological landscape; inconsistencies that are normally very different from and much more concrete than the inconsistencies other people have tried to point out to the client. The client will also start to speak with less fear and fewer psychotic distortions about his or her experiences with the significant persons in their life. This, of course, does not happen in dialogues that sometimes amount to a battle over whose conception of reality is the correct one. Occasionally, clients diagnosed with psychosis have expressed to me that they feel our conversations are little oases of safety and freedom to express themselves, contrasting our talks, implicitly or explicitly, with all the reality correction they are exposed to in their talks with other people. This is not surprising from a person-centred point of view, since reality correction is, basically, an expression of negative regard for the client's own perception of reality.

The points I have made above are also in accordance with Rogers' concept of the fully functioning person (Rogers, 1959, pp. 234–5) that it takes quite a high degree of openness to one's experiences to receive corrections of one's conception of reality non-defensively. Such openness to one's experiences is certainly not what normally characterises people diagnosed with psychosis; often it is quite the opposite.

The dialogue with Svend in my previous chapter pp. 70–2, this volume is an example of a typical transition from expression of relatively more to relatively less psychotic ideation in the course of a person-centred therapy session where, of course, no effort at reality correction is made. It illustrates that expressions of empathic understanding (and the contact reflections of Pre-Therapy that characterise the first part of the session) are in no way reinforcing of psychotic ideation, quite the reverse.

The confusion of 'non-directive' with 'unstructured'

It is common in psychiatric circles to believe that patients diagnosed with psychosis need 'structure'. What is meant by 'structure', though, is rarely defined. The practical implications of the conviction that psychotic patients need structure is normally that an appropriate psychotherapeutic approach is assumed to be one that is goal directed and where the therapist structures the process by trying to keep the client's focus on a certain issue or on several issues in an ordered sequence. In my experience some clients feel helped by this rather patronising approach, others don't, but this has nothing to do with whether or not they belong to the 'worried well' group.

As a consequence of the belief that seriously distressed clients and particularly clients diagnosed with a psychotic condition need 'structure', the non-directive attitude of the person-centred therapist is thought of as being potentially harmful, as a passive laissez-faire attitude that leaves the client helpless in his or her world of hallucinations and delusions or other distressing experiences. What this view ignores is the potency of the core conditions to create a safe and reliable atmosphere for the client and thus what is missed is the most important aspect of the notion of 'structure', the reliability of the social environment of a person. At the difficult edge clients are, in my experience, more vulnerable than people at large to surprises in the way their significant others relate with them. In this sense I think it is true that clients at the difficult edge need structure. They seem to thrive better (and be a little further away from a difficult edge) when they know rather precisely what they can expect of others and when expectations have once been established, if these are not disappointed or nullified at a later time. One could also say that they, more than most other people, seem to need others to relate consistently (or congruently) with them.

In this sense, person-centred therapy is probably the most structured approach of all psychotherapeutic approaches. Any client, including clients diagnosed with psychosis, quickly learns what they can expect from their person-centred therapist: the therapist's very best effort at unconditionally acceptant empathic understanding. This is the consistent attitude of the therapist all through the course of therapy; the person-centred therapist doesn't change attitude in sudden and surprising – and thereby, to the most distressed clients, potentially provocative or over-stimulating – ways.

The person-centred therapist's non-directive attitude is, of course, a direct consequence of the therapist's very active effort at following the client's process with acceptant empathic understanding. There is nothing passive or laissez faire about it, no unstructured letting the client down, or leaving the client to his or her own devices, isolated and unaccompanied. It is truly unfortunate and sad that the therapist's non-directive attitude in person-centred therapy has been misunderstood in this way, and to the degree 'non-directive' is confused with 'unstructured' it is particularly unfortunate and sad for clients at the difficult edge, because this confusion is one of the reasons person-centred therapy has been dismissed as unsuitable for these people, when the truth is, in my experience, that it is eminently suitable for them (see Sommerbeck, 2003).

The erroneous notion that person-centred therapy is too in-depth and exploratory

In some circles, at least in many psychiatric circles, person-centred therapy is regarded as an in-depth exploratory approach on a par with psychodynamic therapy. The majority of professionals in psychiatry assume that an exploratory approach would not benefit their clients or, worse, that an exploratory approach is likely to be harmful to them.

In my experience it is true that people in psychotic or near-psychotic conditions are easily harmed by an in-depth exploratory approach that, more or less subtly, directs the client to still deeper levels of experiencing, and to still closer contact with emotionally stimulating material. The therapist who is biased towards 'deep is better than shallow' and 'close is better than distant' and therefore more or less systematically aims in the direction of 'deeper' and 'closer' does pose a risk to psychotic clients who can easily be overwhelmed and over-stimulated by what is normally regarded as 'deep' and 'close'. People in psychotic or near-psychotic conditions tend to respond to feeling overwhelmed and over-stimulated by displaying more rather than less so-called psychotic behaviours.

To the degree this bias ('deep' is better than 'shallow' and 'close' is better than 'distant') is shared by person-centred therapists, their approach may indeed be harmful to some 'difficult edge' clients. Unfortunately this bias exists for some therapists of *any* orientation, perhaps as a consequence of working with less-disturbed clients in private practice, university clinics, out-patient clinics, etc. If therapists work predominantly with clients who have never set foot in a psychiatric hospital and never will, the notion that 'deep and close is better than shallow and distant' is probably inconsequential and may even be helpful.

The existence of this bias among person-centred therapists is illustrated with the notion, described by some influential authors, that 'additive empathy' (Mearns & Thorne, 1999, p. 45) or empathic understanding of 'edge of awareness experiences' (ibid., p. 52) are preferable to accurate empathy with what the client, in this moment, wants the therapist to understand about his or her psychological landscape. If this understanding of Mearns and Thorne is correct, the person-centred therapist should, according to these authors, aim at additive empathy and empathy with edge of awareness experiences as opposed to 'ordinary' accurate empathic understanding of the client's inner frame of reference or psychological landscape. This preference is, apparently, supported by research, for example, Rainer Sachse (1990, pp. 300–2) has shown that clients typically react with a deepening of their level of experience when the therapist systematically strives for 'deep' empathic understanding responses and succeeds in this. However, the clients in this research were ambulatory clients, not in-patients in a psychiatric hospital. In-patients in a psychiatric hospital are, of course, more seriously psychologically disturbed, probably psychotic or in a so-called borderline condition, and they will typically react with withdrawal and/or intensification of psychotic symptoms to any effort to direct them to deeper levels of experiencing, whether it be by aiming systematically at additive empathy or empathy with edge of awareness experiences or by any other means. The tacit assumption that a deepening of the level of experiencing during the session is synonymous with therapeutic progress is not true for clients in psychotic or near-psychotic conditions.

More recently the notion of working at 'relational depth' (Mearns & Cooper, 2005) has become popular among person-centred practitioners. The helpfulness of aiming at relational depth is, however, likewise questionable when working with clients in psychotic or near-psychotic conditions.

Therapist efforts at directing the client towards deeper levels of experiencing are, of course, in-depth exploratory approaches. Rogers offers the following caution about such in-depth exploratory approaches:

> In the freedom of therapy, as the individual expresses more and more of himself, he finds himself on the verge of voicing a feeling which is obviously and undeniably true, but which is flatly contradictory to the conception of himself which he has held. ... Anxiety results, and if the situation is appropriate [a later section discloses that this means that the core conditions are dominant (this author's comment)], this anxiety is moderate, and the result is constructive. But if, through overzealous and effective interpretation by the therapist, or through some other means, the individual is brought face to face with more of his denied experiences than he can handle, disorganization ensues and a psychotic break occurs. (Rogers, 1959, pp. 229–30)

Raskin (1988, p. 33) eloquently differentiates between systematic and unsystematic therapist responses and says that therapists making systematic responses have '... a preconceived notion of how they wish to change the client and work at it in systematic fashion, in contrast to the person-centered therapist who starts out being open and remains open to an emerging process orchestrated by the client'.

Aiming systematically at additive empathy or empathy of edge of awareness experiences or relational depth can, in my experience, be precisely such an overzealous intervention that can easily bring seriously distressed and disturbed clients face to face with more of their denied experiences than they can handle.

The usefulness of person-centred therapy to clients diagnosed with psychosis or other forms of severe psychopathology hinges, precisely, on the non-directive attitude of the therapist with respect to content as well as to direction of the process. Psychotic clients, and clients with a 'borderline' diagnoses (and many other clients, as the chapters of this book demonstrate, see, for example, Chapter 4 by Peter Pearce and Ros Sewell, this volume), will often flatten their level of experiencing, as a sort of healthy recuperation, before they deepen it again. These clients can therefore talk about the latest fashion in shoes in one moment, only to talk about exceedingly painful experiences the next, and the therapist should follow the client in both directions with equal interest and respect.

The following example (factual content has been changed for reasons of confidentiality) illustrates how the therapist follows the client up and down the levels of experiencing with no effort to direct the client to a deeper level of experiencing.[1]

The client was diagnosed with a borderline condition with paranoid features and was admitted to hospital after a suicide attempt that was his reaction to his first-ever girlfriend breaking up their relationship. Formally he is a voluntary client, but a lot of pressure was put on him, by his father and his GP, to make him accept hospitalisation and it was also after a lot of persuasion from staff members that he has started to see the therapist. In the session from which the excerpt is taken, he has been considering the possibility of writing a letter to his girlfriend when he stops talking and looks down on the floor, his face turned a little away from the therapist. The therapist has no idea of what is going on in him, and remains silent. Finally, he looks up and evidently focuses his gaze on some photos on the wallboard in the therapist's office.

> Therapist: You look at the photos.
>
> Client: Yes, is it your dog?
>
> T: Yes.
>
> C: It looks sweet.
>
> T: It is very sweet.
>
> C: It's a beagle, isn't it? [Seemingly pleased that he knows.]
>
> T: Yes ... feel pleased to be able to recognise it?
>
> C: Yes ...We used to have a basset; I did a lot of obedience training with him. Have you done that?
>
> T: Oh, yes, if you don't do that with a beagle, it is just all over the place.
>
> C: [Laughing] Just like with a basset. [Falling silent again, and looking down on the floor. Then he looks at the therapist.]
>
> C: Do you know what incest is?
>
> T: I know what the word means, but I'm not quite sure if that is what you

1. This example first appeared in Sommerbeck, L (2003) *The Client-Centred Therapist in Psychiatric Contexts: A therapists' guide to the psychiatric landscape and its inhabitants*. Ross-on-Wye: PCCS Books.

are asking me?

C: [Quickly looking away from the therapist and down on the floor again.] Yes ... No, incest is many things, isn't it?

T: Yes. [The therapist feels that she has lost contact with Johnny again.]

[Client remains motionless and silent for a while; then he looks out of the window.]

T: You look out of the window.

C: Yes, [looking at the therapist again] aren't you disturbed by all that noise from the birds? [A colony of crows in the big trees outside.]

T: No, not really, I'm so used to them, I seldom notice.

C: You know, I ... I don't know ... that question about incest ... I don't know.

T: There is something about incest bothering you, and maybe it is too hard to talk about?

C: Yes. [Falls silent, seemingly thoughtful.]

C: [Very quickly and abruptly, almost spitting it out] It is about my father and maybe it was incest, I don't know, I don't want to talk about it.

T: You just want me to know that you are troubled by something your father has done that maybe was incest, and you don't want to go into any details about it?

C: [With evident relief] Right, maybe later, I just wanted you to know that this is part of the picture, too.

T: It's a relief that I know there are such things bothering you, too, and that you are not obliged to tell me any details about it?

C: A huge relief and maybe we can talk more about it next time?

T: We sure can.

After a short silence, the client turned to other, much less emotionally provocative and more 'shallow' subjects. He didn't return to the issue of incest until three sessions later, when he associated to the topic after having told how he had had to give up his plan of watching television in the lounge, because the only seat left was next to a male nurse on a small sofa.

The approach of the therapist in this excerpt is non-directive both with respect to content and with respect to process. The therapist does not aim to deepen the client's level of experience by systematically responding with additive empathy or empathy for edge of awareness experiences and the therapist does not aim for relational depth by challenging the client's frequent preference for 'small talk'. The client is in full charge of the direction of the process towards flattening or deepening his level of experience, and the therapist follows the client with equal interest and acceptance in talking about client experiences of dogs and birds as in talking about client experiences of incest. This therapist's approach is, clearly, not an in-depth exploratory approach and it is, therefore, not a potentially harmful approach with people diagnosed with severe psychopathology – on the contrary, as I have already stated.

The confusion of the theory of therapy with the theory of personality

Rogers explains psychopathology as the result of more or less excessive exposure to conditions of worth (see, for example, Rogers, 1959). Contemporary psychiatry, on the contrary, favours biological explanations, particularly for the more serious psychological disturbances (i.e., the disturbances of people diagnosed with a psychotic or near-psychotic condition). If it is assumed that a strongly held belief in the truth of Rogers' theory of personality, including his explanatory theory of psychopathology, is a necessary prerequisite for practising person-centred therapy, then it is also true that person-centred therapy cannot be considered useful with the clients of 'heavy psychiatry' (i.e., work with people with severe and enduring mental health problems). At least not when viewed from the point of view of heavy psychiatry, and when viewed from the point of view of those person-centred therapists who regard Rogers' explanation of psychopathology as the infallible truth, there will be a battle of 'who is right' within psychiatry.

It is my contention, however, that one does not need to be convinced of the truth of Rogers' explanatory theory of psychopathology in order to practise person-centred therapy. One only has to be convinced of the potency of the core conditions and that offering the core conditions to a client is the best one can do, as a psychotherapist, to facilitate actualisation of the client's most constructive potentials. The actualisation of these constructive potentials may have been blocked for a variety of reasons, or the potentials, as such, may have been diminished permanently for a variety of reasons. The reasons may be biological, psychological, cultural, or whatever, but this is of no real consequence to the actual practice of person-centred therapy.

In this connection it is important not to regard person-centred therapy as a curative treatment on a par with medical model treatments. People with severe somatic illnesses or handicaps can benefit from person-centred therapy in the sense that they find better ways to live with their illness or handicap; they do not benefit in the sense that they are cured of their illness or handicap. This is, to a certain degree, also the case with many clients diagnosed with a psychotic condition. Person-centred therapy is useful to them, but not in the sense that they are cured of a presumed biological disposition to process stressful events in psychotic ways, but rather in the sense that they become better able to protect themselves against stress factors that used to release a psychotic breakdown. With these clients, person-centred therapy can be regarded as a preventive, rather than curative, treatment.

On the other hand, it is also true in my experience that many psychotic conditions originate in early traumatic experiences and in these cases person-centred therapy can, indeed, effectuate a cure in the ordinary sense of this word.

There exists, in my experience, no theory that in a fully satisfying way explains the existence of the so-called psychotic conditions, particularly those of schizophrenia and bipolar disorder. It is even doubtful that these conditions do exist as discrete illnesses. I do not believe that Rogers' explanatory theory of psychopathology (excessive exposure to conditions of worth) is the full story of how psychological disturbances come about, although I think it goes a long way in that direction. I think that other factors play a role, too: socio-economic factors, educational factors and, of course, cultural factors that are important for the definition of what a given culture regards as psychopathological behaviour. Finally, I can't disregard what to me seems to be convincing evidence that biological factors play a role too, although in my opinion they play a much more peripheral role than they are given by biologically oriented psychiatrists. Taken together, I think that the factors which determine what the psychiatry of Western societies regard as psychopathological behaviour are as many as they are complexly intertwined.

Thus, confusing Rogers' theory of therapy with Rogers' theory of personality by regarding a strongly held belief in the latter to be a prerequisite for practising the former propagates the myth, at least in psychiatric circles, that person-centred therapy is not useful for clients diagnosed with conditions that are, in these circles, regarded as predominantly biologically determined, particularly the conditions diagnosed as schizophrenia and bipolar disorder. Indeed exactly the opposite is true in my experience: even clients regarded as being beyond psychotherapeutic reach are not beyond the reach of person-centred therapy, particularly when it is extended with Pre-Therapy (Prouty, 1994).

Reaching the unreachable

It is common practice in other schools of psychotherapy to regard people with the most severe psychological disturbances as being beyond psychotherapeutic reach. The basic reason for this is that these therapeutic approaches normally demand some degree of cooperation from the potential client apart from this person allowing the therapist to make a 'perceived or subceived difference' (Rogers, 1959, p. 207) in his/her experiential field. At the very least, therapists of other approaches depend on experiencing a minimal degree of client interest in and ability to:

1. keep a sustained focus of attention
2. make him- or herself understood by the therapist
3. change something about him- or herself and
4. receive and process input/interventions from the therapist's frame.

For various reasons, though, therapists will not have these experiences with many of the clients in the back wards of psychiatry. Floridly psychotic clients rarely keep a sustained focus for any substantial length of time; withdrawn, so-called autistic, clients seem without any wish that others understand anything about them; people diagnosed with delusions of persecution apparently don't feel in need of help to change anything about themselves – they feel in need of having the relevant authorities put a halt to the persecution. People diagnosed with delusions of grandiosity seem to think that it is everyone else who is in need of their help, not the other way around; people diagnosed with a psychotic depression seem so depleted of energy and hope that they can't participate in anything in a therapeutic relationship; and finally, people diagnosed with a manic psychosis feel happily elated without any worries they might wish a therapist's help with. And the groups mentioned are all either incapable of, or uninterested in, receiving input/ interventions from the therapist's frame. Since these are people whose behaviour is often within the area of the application of laws for the use of force in psychiatry, they are frequently involuntarily admitted to hospital and involuntarily treated with medicine. Offers of help from psychiatry that they are allowed to be free to refuse, such as, for example, psychotherapy, they normally do refuse.

Of course, this list is a crude generalisation. It is stereotypical and leaves out all the nuances and degrees in these peoples' variations with respect to the stereotype. Still, in these stereotypes lie the reasons these clients are normally considered beyond psychotherapeutic reach. They are, however, not beyond the reach of person-centred therapy, often in combination with Pre-Therapy.

In my experience, the reason for this is the non-directive attitude of the person-centred therapist. This therapist makes no particular interventions in the hope that they will be helpful to the client. Of course, the therapist hopes that the relationship, in general, will benefit the client, but in a very basic sense he or she meets the client with an offer of interest rather than with an offer of help. The therapist tries to experience the client's momentary psychological landscape as the client experiences it; he or she has no wish to change the client in any way, only to get to know the client to the degree the client allows it. The clients described above are usually hypersensitive to other people's wishes to change them, and when they sense such wishes in another they typically react with resistance and withdrawal. They do not normally resist or withdraw, though, when they are approached with a sincere interest in who they are and where they are as an individual. In this case they may put a limit to the contact because they have better things to do than being with the therapist, not because they are resistive or fearful of the contact, as such. And in many cases, they welcome the therapist's interest and some end up wishing the contact to continue because they feel helped by it and want further help. At this point the relationship has developed into an ordinary client-centred therapy relationship that is motivated by the client's wish for help as much, or more, than by the therapist's interest in the client.

It is, thus, not only a myth that person-centred therapy is not useful with clients diagnosed with severe psychopathology. It is the opposite of the truth.

Person-centred therapy is eminently suited for these clients and with the extension of Pre-Therapy, person-centred therapy can reach clients in the most remote corners of the back wards of psychiatry. Psychiatric nurses, who have participated in training groups in Pre-Therapy that I have facilitated, do not, as is normally the case, ask: 'Is this client too disturbed to benefit from the approach?' On the contrary, they ask: 'Is this client too little disturbed to benefit from the approach?' I feel touched by this, because it is evidence, to me, that finally an approach has been found that makes it possible to reach the unreachable, an approach for those who are worst off, not another approach for those who are best off.

References

Mearns, D & Thorne, B (1999) *Person-Centred Counselling in Action*. London: Sage.

Mearns, D & Cooper, M (2005) *Working at Relational Depth in Counselling and Psychotherapy*. London: Sage.

Prouty, G (1994) *Theoretical Evolutions in Person-Centered/Experiential Therapy: Applications to schizophrenic and retarded psychoses*. Westport, CT: Praeger.

Prouty, G, Van Werde, D & Pörtner, M (2002) *Pre-Therapy: Reaching contact-impaired clients*. Ross-on-Wye: PCCS Books.

Raskin, N (1988) *What Do We Mean by Person-Centered Therapy?* Paper presented at the second meeting of the Association for the Development of the Person-Centered Approach, New York.

Rogers, CR (1959) A theory of therapy, personality, and interpersonal relationships as developed in the client-centered framework. In E Koch (Ed) *Psychology: A study of a science, Vol. 3: Formulations of the person and the social context* (pp. 184–256). New York: McGraw-Hill.

Sachse, R (1990) Concrete interventions are crucial: The influence of the therapist's processing proposals on the client's intrapersonal exploration in client-centered therapy. In G Lietaer, J Rombauts, and R Van Balen (Eds) *Client-Centered and Experiential Psychotherapy in the Nineties* (pp. 295–308). Leuven, Belgium: Leuven University Press.

Sanders, P (Ed) (2007) *The Contact Work Primer: An introduction to Pre-Therapy and the work of Garry Prouty*. Ross-on-Wye: PCCS Books.

Sommerbeck, L (2003) *The Client-Centred Therapist in Psychiatric Contexts: A therapists' guide to the psychiatric landscape and its inhabitants*. Ross-on-Wye: PCCS Books.

Vitger, J (1999) Kurative Faktorer ved Psykoanalytiske Terapier. *Matrix*, 3, 200.

Therapist limits at the difficult edge | **13**

Lisbeth Sommerbeck

At the difficult edge, therapist limits are frequently challenged. Actually, this can be regarded as one way of understanding the term 'the difficult edge': the difficulty is in the eye of the beholder, in the therapist's experience when getting to the edge or limit of his or her capacity. The limits may be limits of competence with respect to empathic understanding and unconditional acceptance of the client, the limits may be more or less idiosyncratic, or the limits may be those inherent, explicitly or implicitly, in the context the therapist is working in. The scope of this chapter does not allow discussion of the latter kind of limits – interested readers are referred to Sommerbeck, 2012.

The chapter represents the sum of my experience with these issues, the experience of a long career within a psychiatric context where a large part of the therapeutic work takes place at the 'difficult edge'.

Limits of therapeutic competence

The central competence of person-centred therapists is their capacity to congruently experience unconditional positive regard for, and empathic understanding of, the client. At the difficult edge, however, a therapist can easily reach their limit in this capacity. We shall first discuss limits in the experience of empathic understanding of the client and then proceed to consider limits in the experience of unconditional positive regard for the client. It should be remembered that in practice this is ordinarily *one* experience. It is only in theory and for clarity's sake that this experience can be separated into empathic understanding on the one hand and unconditional positive regard on the other hand. An analogy for this could be that, in practice, water cannot be separated into oxygen and hydrogen even if it makes sense to discuss these elements separately.

Limits in the therapist's experience of empathic understanding

1. When feeling out of contact with the client

Rogers said (1959, p. 210) that 'being empathic is to perceive the *internal* frame of reference of another with accuracy ...' (my italics). Thus, empathic understanding means that one understands something of what goes on *beneath* the skin of the client. However, at the difficult edge therapists often experience clients as being 'out of contact', meaning that they have no idea what goes on beneath the skin of the client, no idea of the client's *inner* world or internal frame of reference. Instead, clients appear withdrawn, monologising or emotionally overwhelmed. In these conditions clients are unable to, or uninterested in, making themselves understood by the therapist, who therefore misses a sense of empathic mutuality with the client. The most likely impact of this is that the therapist will feel at a loss and rather helpless as far as empathic understanding of the client is concerned. As therapists we can easily feel we have come to the limit of our capacity on such occasions, because we find ourselves unable to do what we are most used to and most practised at doing: understanding the client empathically.

Garry Prouty's seminal contribution was, precisely, the development of a therapeutic mode, 'Pre-Therapy', that allows therapists to relate to clients in a truly person-centred way when the therapist's capacity for empathic understanding of the *inner* frame of reference of the client fails (Prouty, 1994; Prouty, Van Werde & Pörtner, 2002). The reason for this is that the so-called contact reflections of Pre-Therapy are attuned to the observable surface, not to the internal frame of reference of the client. They are attuned to the observable facial expressions, bodily gestures, words and immediate situational surroundings of the client and not to what may be going on beneath the skin of the client as is the case with ordinary empathic responses.

Before I learned about Pre-Therapy, I knew there were clients in the back wards of psychiatric institutions that I was unable to work with. It was a great joy to become able to approach these clients in a pre-therapeutic way, to know that there were no longer clients who were beyond (my) therapeutic reach, at least not for reasons of limits of empathic understanding.

The practice of Pre-Therapy is described in more detail in Chapter 6 on pp. 67–73 and will therefore not be further explicated here – for more detailed descriptions see Prouty, Van Werde and Pörtner, 2002 and Sanders, 2007.

2. When being the target of extreme affects

At the difficult edge, clients frequently experience and express relatively extreme affects towards the therapist, and whether they are positive or negative they can be a particular challenge to the therapist's capacity for empathic understanding.

This is so because therapists can easily become overly emotionally involved in these situations or, on the contrary, withdraw their emotional involvement in the interaction with the client. In the first case, accuracy of empathic understanding can tend to be diminished when 'tainted' with the therapist's own emotional response; in the latter case, expressions of empathic understanding can tend to become mechanical, wooden and 'parrot like'.

In such cases, client emotions expressed more or less subtly often lie along a dimension that might be described as devaluation–idealisation. On the one hand, clients might mock and ridicule the therapist, particularly the therapist's competence, in a way that can get under the skin of even the most experienced therapist, who then may feel more or less defensive or valueless. On the other, clients can also express extreme admiration for the therapist, who can then have a hard time not 'falling for it' and starting to believe that he or she is indispensable for the client; the only one who is able to understand and help them. Alternatively, the therapist may feel awkward with all this praise, almost ashamed of empathising with it in its full degree and instead tend toward inserting a measure of modesty with a sobering response to the client.

In my experience, no therapist, however experienced and competent, is immune to reactions along these lines when on the receiving end of such extreme emotions. With clients who express devaluation of them, therapists can help themselves by remembering all the clients who have been helped by these qualities of relating, and with clients who express idealisation of them, therapists might help themselves by remembering how some of their former idealising clients actually idealised others too. They might hold their awkwardness at bay by remembering that empathic understanding is not only understanding of the content but also of the intensity and extremeness of emotions. However, when working at the difficult edge, these 'rules of thumb' cannot stand alone. Peer support and consultation is, in my opinion, a necessity in order to avoid getting stuck or tangled up in relationships with emotionally extreme clients that become less and less therapeutic – relationships where therapists might increasingly lose sight both of original intentions and respect for their own limits and instead feel increasingly burdened and restricted in their relationship with the client.

Like everybody else, therapists fluctuate in their level of competence and these fluctuations tend to be more marked when working at the difficult edge. Sometimes the therapist's work is absolutely brilliant, sometimes it is pretty far below his or her ordinary level. Rogers' own practice was no exception to this: the following two examples of dialogue show Rogers responding, first, to a very aggressively devaluating client, who seems to be on the brink of psychosis, with, in my opinion, beautiful warmth and accuracy of empathic understanding. In the second example, however, he appears rather withdrawn and mechanical in his responses to a client (from the Wisconsin project,[1] diagnosed with schizophrenia) who mocks and ridicules his competence in a subtler and more composed way than the first, which may have made it harder to work with.

> Client: [... begins to talk in hard flat voice, quite unlike her usual tone. Does not look at counselor ...] You feel I want to come, but I don't! I'm not coming anymore. It doesn't do any good. I don't like you. I hate you! I wish you were never born.
>
> Rogers: You just hate me very bitterly.
>
> Client: I think I'll throw you in the lake. I'll cut you up! You think people like you, but they don't ... You think you can attract women but you can't ... I wish you were *dead*.
>
> Rogers: You detest me and you'd really like to get rid of me.
>
> Client: You think my father did bad things with me, but he didn't! You think he wasn't a good man, but he *was*. You think I want intercourse but I *don't*.
>
> Rogers: You feel that I *absolutely misrepresent* all your thoughts.
>
> Client: ... You think you can get people to come in and tell you everything, and they'll think they're being helped, but they're *not*. You just like to make 'em suffer. You think you can hypnotize them, but you *can't*! You think you're good, but you ain't. I hate you. I *hate* you.
>
> Rogers: You feel I really like to make 'em suffer, but I don't help them.
>
> Client: You think I haven't been straight, but I have. I *hate* you. All I've had is pain, pain, pain. You think I can't direct my own life, but I can. You think I can't get well, but I can. You think I had hallucinations, but I didn't. I hate you. [Long pause, leans on desk in strained, exhausted pose] You think I'm crazy but I'm not.
>
> Rogers: You're sure I think you're crazy.
>
> Client: [Pause] I'm tired, and I just can't get loose! [Despairing tone of voice and tears. Pause.] I had a hallucination and I've got to get it out! ... [Goes on about her deep conflicts, and tells of her hallucination she has experienced with terrific tension in her voice, but with an attitude very different from that at the beginning of the interview.]
>
> [Later in interview]
>
> Client: I knew at the office I had to get rid of this somewhere. I felt I could come down and tell you. I knew you'd understand. I couldn't say I hated myself. That's true but I couldn't say it. So I just thought of all the ugly things I could say to you instead.
>
> Rogers: The things you felt about yourself you couldn't say, but you could say them to me.
>
> Client: I know we're coming to rock bottom. (Rogers, 1951, pp. 211–13)

---

1. In 1957 Rogers became director of the Psychology and Psychiatry departments at Wisconsin University. Here he and his co-workers engaged in a large research project to study client-centred therapy with people diagnosed with schizophrenia (Rogers et al., 1967). The reasons for the somewhat disappointing results have been analysed by Sommerbeck (2002).

In a footnote Rogers writes:

> Just as it is impossible to convey on paper the venom and hatred in the client's voice, so it is utterly impossible to convey the depth of empathy in the counselor's [Rogers'] responses. The counselor states, 'I tried to enter into and to express in my voice the full degree of soul-consuming anger which she was pouring out. The written words look incredibly pale, but in the situation they were full of the same feeling she was so coldly and deeply expressing.' (1951, p. 212)

And, evidently, this was a very fruitful interview at a very difficult edge.

The second example is taken from a transcript available from the Carl Rogers Memorial Library at the Center for Studies of the Person, La Jolla, California. The title of it is 'Carl Rogers' reconstruction of his first Wisconsin case'. The client did not allow the interviews to be recorded, so the transcript is based on the notes Rogers wrote after the sessions.

> [From the fifth interview]
>
> Client: Have you had experience working with people where drinking is the problem?
>
> [Long pause]
>
> Rogers: I'm trying to sort of see what my feelings are in response to that. The factual answer to your question is easy enough. The factual answer is simply, 'some'. But I also find myself feeling something beyond that. The feeling is, I am just whatever I am in this relationship.
>
> Client: What does that mean?
>
> Rogers: I guess it means nothing to you, so let's skip it.
>
> Client: You kind of put me on the defensive. I feel as though it isn't right somehow for me to ask questions of you – as though you aren't willing for me or don't want me to ask you questions. And yet these questions are vital to me.
>
> Rogers: I guess it seems to you that somehow I'm not really receptive to the things you want to ask and yet they're damned significant to you.

There follow some exchanges about their mutual lack of knowledge about each other and then the fifth interview ends as follows:

> Client: You say you don't know anything of me. You're ignorant of me. You're ignorant about me. You don't seem to want to take any steps to remedy that ignorance. I don't know you. I'm ignorant about you. How could anything happen in a situation like that?
>
> Rogers: I guess you feel that it's kind of an impasse which has similarities on both sides. I have no knowledge of you. I don't seem to be taking action to remedy that. You feel equally lacking in knowledge about me: and so how could anything come of it?

> Client: I say something my way, and then you say it your way. It's just fascinating that I try to say something and then you put it in your words. It's just like an echo chamber.
>
> [Long pause]
>
> Rogers: I see our time is up for today. Friday?
>
> Client [After long pause] Put up or shut up. [Long pause] Okay.

From the seventh and last interview [the client had actually wished to stop seeing Rogers, but Rogers had asked him to come for this interview]:

> Client: I don't understand why I'm here this morning.
>
> Rogers: As far as I'm concerned, I simply asked if you would come and you have come and I appreciate that.
>
> Client: I've done you a favor, is that it?
>
> Rogers: Yes, and I appreciate it.
>
> Client: So you're obligated to me?
>
> Rogers: No, I feel no sense of obligation. I asked you to come in, you did, and I appreciated it; I told you things I wanted to express to you.
>
> Client: Then you feel no sense of obligation?
>
> Rogers: No.
>
> Client: Do you know anything more about me than you did when I last saw you?
>
> Rogers: No, would you like me to?
>
> Client: I won't answer that.
>
> Rogers: I must seem to you like a pretty strange duck, not even finding out about you from the record and so on.
>
> Client: No, you're not strange; I find you very usual ... Well, I've done my favor, I guess I can go.
>
> Rogers: I appreciate your coming in, and I would like to see you a week from today at this same time if you're willing, so that we can get together for several casual contacts, so that we could get to know each other better in order that in time you could really decide whether you wanted to continue it or not. You don't need to answer that now, however, unless you wish.
>
> Client: I'm willing to answer that now, and the answer is no.

The client got up to leave the room and Rogers said 'Goodbye' and the client said 'Goodbye'.

I have speculated that this may well be one of the clients Rogers was thinking of when he wrote (Rogers et al., 1967, footnote 2, p. 26) that he regretted not having included a measure for client motivation in the Wisconsin project.

3. When missing a red thread

Most therapists associate empathic understanding with also being able to follow the 'red thread' or a certain degree of logical coherence in the client's narrative. This, of course, means that a red thread is expected, but when working at the difficult edge, there will often be an apparent lack of such a red thread. The only remedy is to lower one's expectations in terms of being able to follow the client's narrative. The client may seem to jump incomprehensibly from one point to another and in this case it is important that therapists have great tolerance for their own 'not-understanding'. The therapist will understand in bits and pieces, but they must tolerate that they cannot see any connection between these bits and pieces. What the client says can seem very fragmented, and in following this, the therapist's responses will be fragmented too – one response feels unassociated with the preceding one and from the next to come. Therapy with these clients is an exercise par excellence in 'holding and letting go'. It is important that the therapist does not hold on to the understanding of one moment in order to save his or her own sense of continuity, but lets go of this understanding in order to follow the client's next move, even if it seems contradictory to the one preceding it. Such a position is echoed in Rogers' writing with regard to unconditional positive regard: 'It involves … as much acceptance of ways he [the client] is inconsistent as of ways in which he is consistent' (Rogers, 1957, p. 98).

4. When empathic understanding is difficult to communicate

Work at the difficult edge also means that the therapist can meet clients who monologise in a fast, seemingly endless, stream of associations, apparently under a huge pressure to talk. If the therapist wants to do his or her job of following and understanding empathically with these clients, it can be necessary to interrupt the client's stream of talking quite forcefully with 'Wait a minute, let me see if I have understood you …', or something to the same effect. If therapists do not do this, they will in all likelihood be left totally behind and, in the process, come to feel increasingly out of contact with the client. On the contrary, in my experience therapists will experience an increase in their sense of mutuality in the contact with the client by insisting on doing their job of trying to understand. They will also experience an increase in the client's interest in the contact, as if these clients slowly realise that the therapist truly wants to understand them, that the therapist is not out to correct them, silence them or whatever. Interrupting the fast-streaming monologues of clients in this way may superficially seem like a violation of the principle of non-directivity, but on a deeper level it means that the therapist stays with the client, that the client is not left alone by the therapist giving up trying to follow the client and instead just letting the client's words pass in through one ear and out through the other.

Limits in the therapist's experience of unconditional positive regard

All therapists now and then experience fluctuations in their level of unconditional positive regard for, or unconditional acceptance of, the client and probably this is particularly the case at the difficult edge, often, precisely as an expression of the difficulty of practising at that edge.

An example: With the recent focus on paedophilia and the offering of therapy to paedophiles, a frequent student concern is their sense that it will be impossible for them to experience unconditional positive regard for a paedophile client. They experience a limit that they feel unable to transcend and are also sometimes *unwilling* to transcend out of sheer abhorrence of the particular crime of paedophilia. In the latter case, they should of course not get into work with paedophiles, but in the former case there are ways of thinking that can promote unconditional positive regard for the paedophile, as well as for other clients whose behaviour one tends to distance oneself sharply from.

It is, for example, often said that unconditional acceptance is for the essential humaneness of the client, not for the behaviour of the client. In this vein, Barrett-Lennard (1998, p. 66) says that limit setting is 'on behaviour, not on attitudes and feelings'. Rogers, however, seemed doubtful about this. He wrote (Rogers et al., 1967, pp. 103–4):

> The question is often raised: but what about the therapist's attitude toward his client's asocial or antisocial behavior? Is he to accept this without evaluation? Sometimes this question is answered by saying that the effective therapist prizes the person, but not necessarily his behavior. Yet it is doubtful if this is an adequate or true answer. To be sure, the therapist may feel that a particular behavior is socially unacceptable or socially bad, something he could not approve of in himself, and a way of behaving which is inimical to the welfare of the social group. But the effective therapist may feel acceptant of this behavior in his client, not as desirable behavior, but as a *natural consequence* of the circumstances, experiences, and feelings of this client. Thus the therapist's acceptance may be based upon this kind of feeling: 'If I had had the same background, the same circumstances, the same experiences, it would be inevitable in me, as it is in this client, that I would act in this fashion.' ...
>
> Thus when the therapist prizes his client, and is searching for the meaning or value of his client's thoughts or behaviors within the client, he does not tend to feel a response of approval or disapproval. He feels an acceptance of what *is*.

This quotation has made much sense to me, and been very helpful for me when I experienced a decrease in my unconditional acceptance of the client. Let me give a striking example from my own practice:

The day after the 9/11 attacks on the US, my colleagues and I of course shared our horror at these events at our ordinary 'morning briefing' the next day. We had all been sitting glued to the television until the very late – or very early – hours of the night. We agreed that we all felt a need to mark this sad day by raising the flag to half-mast on the lawn outside and keep a minute's silence while doing so. In this mood of sadness we separated to start the day's work. I went to my office to meet with my first client that day. As she entered the room, she looked out of the window and exclaimed: 'But the flag shouldn't be at half-mast! It should be all up! This is a wonderful day; now America has been taught the lesson it has deserved for ages; it is a reason for jubilation, not for sadness' – and more to the same effect. And she spoke in the same rather shrill tone of voice that I had heard on television the night before when I in horror had witnessed the scenes of jubilation in the streets of Gaza.

I was completely taken aback and while she spoke, my previous acceptance of her changed to loathing – I actually felt like throwing her out of the room! And I was close to panicking, feeling like this, feeling so utterly anti-therapeutic, and I toyed for some seconds with the idea of excusing myself and cancelling our session, because of a sudden headache or other excuse. Then I took a very firm grip on myself, telling myself that I was not supposed to be a judge of her, nor a political discussion partner, nor a teacher, nor anything but her therapist, and that that meant trying to understand her empathically. All this whirled around in my mind in a matter of seconds, so when we settled down in our chairs, I was firmly decided on putting my own perspective as far away as possible in favour of concentrating on hers. In the first minutes of the session this was no small feat; I was not nearly as present in our interaction as normally and my empathic understanding responses were certainly rather 'wooden'. Nevertheless, she responded with further exploration of her experience, and consequently, as Rogers wrote, I did indeed start to understand more of the meaning and value of her thoughts to her, and to understand how they were a natural consequence of her experiences and her background. In this process my acceptance of her slowly increased to its ordinary level and I could again be fully present with her. My loathing evaporated.

It turned out that her reaction to seeing the flag at half-mast had a lot to do with her very complex relationship with her recently deceased father whom she described as a hard-core communist. He would have loved what had happened, she said, and then she added: 'And I do, too, but I wish the Twin Towers could have crumbled to ashes without anybody dying. All those people dead, all those who will now be missed like I miss my father!' And then she started crying. When she left I was as fond of our relationship as ever and very satisfied with the decision I had made at the start of the session.

In this example, the therapist's diminished acceptance was short lived and empathic understanding relatively quickly increased acceptance to its normal level. However, if the diminution of the therapist's experience of unconditional acceptance turns out to be relatively persistent, it is time for consultation/

supervision, or, as a last resort for many therapists, they may find it necessary to share their experiences with the client in order to 'clear the air in the hope that the client will understand that the experiences of the therapist are the therapist's and do not necessarily reflect on the client. Therapists surely vary in the degree of self-disclosure they find relevant, and in some forms of person-centred therapy, therapist self-disclosures are much more prominent than in others. This is the case, for example, in relational depth therapy compared with classical client-centred therapy, and these probably represent a continuum of 'congruent' self-disclosure.

There is another way of thinking which can be helpful in maintaining the experience of unconditional positive regard for the client. When a therapist likes the interaction with the client, they may have a sense of liking the client and thus unconditional acceptance comes more easily. But this sense of liking the client may be treacherous. It comes naturally when one likes the interaction with the client, but in contexts other than therapy one might not like the interaction with the client and thus not 'like the client' – and the client, in turn, might not 'like the therapist'. What if they were put side by side at a festive dinner? What if the therapist were a student of the client in her job as a history teacher? What if they were to co-work on a building project? In these contexts they might not necessarily like their interaction with each other, and thus they might not have the sense of liking each other. But as far as the therapist's experience of unconditional acceptance of the client goes, it suffices for the therapist to enjoy the interaction with the client in the context of *therapy*, in his or her role as a therapist for this other person in their role as client. Neither therapist nor client can know how they'd feel about each other outside the context of therapy.[2] It is therefore important for therapists that they generally enjoy their work and that they secure, in whatever way possible, their ability to look forward to their next therapy session with the client with appreciation, and securing this has much to do with their success in protecting their experience of therapeutic freedom and comfort in their relationship with the client. All of the previous discussion in this chapter could be said to have the goal of helping therapists to do precisely that, and this is also the case with the discussion of limit setting that follows below.

Generally about limit setting

Surprisingly little has been written in the person-centred literature about limit setting with adult clients, even if it is a topic that most students of person-centred

2. These points are not meant to be a contribution to the discussion of the appropriateness for therapists to engage in extra-therapeutic relationships with their clients. Doing this may often be unethical, or at least ethically arguable. On the other hand, I have had many colleagues among the nursing staff in brief crisis therapy after some violent episode in the ward. At the same time I have been co-working with them as usual, and it has worked fine. It may, of course, make a difference that I enjoyed our (extra-therapeutic) relationship as colleagues *before* we also engaged in a therapeutic relationship.

therapy, as well as experienced practitioners, are concerned with. In order to find a relatively extensive treatment of the subject, I had to go all the way back to Rogers' own book *Counseling and Psychotherapy* (1942), where he devotes a whole section (pp. 95–108) to 'The Matter of Limits'.

Here Rogers writes:

> The amateur or untrained counselor, bolstered by good intentions, anxious not to hurt the client, has a tendency to accede to the requests, to do almost anything which the client feels will help, until the demand upon time or affection or responsibility grow too great for the counselor to bear. Then his affection and desire to help turn to avoidance and dislike. He blames the client and rejects him. The net result is that the client feels that one more person has betrayed him, that one more person who claimed to wish to help has actually failed in time of stress. He may be definitely and sometimes permanently hurt by this bungled attempt at counseling. (p. 96)

In my experience, it is not only inexperienced therapists who can exceed their limits like this. At the difficult edge it can also happen, mostly quite inadvertently and/or imperceptibly, to the experienced therapist. And it is, of course, important that therapists do not end up in the vicious 'saviour/victim/persecutor' triangle that Rogers described in the quotation above.

In *Client-Centred Therapy* (Rogers, 1951, p. 211) there is just a footnote about limit setting:

> As in setting any limit in the therapeutic experience, this is something which is purely the responsibility of the therapist, and he takes that responsibility. He does not attempt to evaluate the client's experience by some such statement as 'That really wouldn't help you'. He simply takes responsibility for his own behavior, at the same time indicating understanding and acceptance of the client's experience of the situation.

This footnote is a comment on an example of limit setting (Rogers, 1951, p. 211), which might be illustrative to include here, as it is also probably characteristic of limit setting in today's person-centred practice:

> Client: I think emotionally I'm dying for sexual intercourse but I don't do anything about it. ... The thing I want is to have sexual intercourse with you. I don't dare ask you, because I'm afraid you'd be nondirective.
>
> Rogers: You have this awful tension, and want so much to have relations with me.
>
> Client [Goes on in the same vein. Finally]: Can't we do something about it? This tension is awful! Will you relieve the tension ... Can you give me a direct answer? I think it might help both of us.
>
> Rogers: [Gently] The answer would be no. I can understand how *desperately* you feel, but I would not be willing to do that.

> Client: [Pause; sigh of relief] I think that helps me. It's only when I'm upset
> that I'm like this. You have strength, and it gives me strength.

In January 2012 I participated in an email network (PCINTL@LISTSERV.UGA.EDU) discussion of person-centred practitioners about limits and limit setting. I received permission from some of the participants to quote them here, as I found their contributions clarifying for today's perspectives on limit setting in person-centred practice. Jin Wu wrote:

> The client-centered therapist checks with oneself to see if honoring a client's request would compromise one's ability to provide the conditions, so such limits vary a great deal from therapist to therapist; one might be able to take 3am phone calls, another might not be able to go 5 minutes longer for the session. In other words, a client-centred therapist has an internal locus of control for setting limits, not necessarily an external standard (beyond what's legal).

Dorothy Morgan wrote:

> I think limits and limit setting would fall within the category of genuineness in that it would be presented as, 'I am unable to follow you there (for whatever reason)'. I do think it is important that limits be presented in terms of an inability of the therapist rather than as correct/incorrect, appropriate/ inappropriate, etc.

Kathy Moon wrote (quoting from her own article on therapy with children (Moon, 2001, pp. 46–7):

> I prefer to say that limits are set in the service of the therapist. The purpose is to help the therapist maintain equanimity and positive regard towards the client. Limits are set in the service of the child only because they are necessary to the therapist in order for the therapist to remain acceptant, empathic and congruent. I consider any other purpose for limits to be didactic and contrary to the condition of unconditional positive regard.

There were other contributions in the same vein, and it thus seems to be a fairly general view that limit setting is for the protection of the therapist's capacity to remain unconditionally acceptant and empathically understanding of the client. Or, put another way, by respecting their own limits therapists avoid getting into the saviour/victim/persecutor triangle in their relationship with clients, where therapists sacrifice their limits in order to save the client, who, to the therapist, appears unable to cope with the therapist's limit, only for the therapist to end up, more or less subtly and unaware, blaming (i.e., a kind of persecuting) the client for his or her ingratitude for their sacrifice and feeling a victim of client demands. In none of these positions can there be any question of unconditional positive regard for the client. Unconditional positive regard for the client can only be experienced when therapists feel free, including free to express their own limits, in their relationship with clients.

Nevertheless, particularly at the difficult edge, therapists now and then end up in this vicious triangle with a client. A way out of it is to apologise to the client for having exceeded one's own limits as soon as one becomes aware that one has, indeed, done so. If this is not done explicitly (admitting to having committed an error with any subsequent explanation and discussion it may entail), the relationship is likely to be harmed by an undercurrent of feelings of regret and restrictions. It is the therapist's responsibility to regain his or her experience of feeling free in the relationship with the client, so that unconditional positive regard for the client can again be experienced.

Will the client reject the therapist?

Rogers wrote (1942, p. 99) about the risk of the client rejecting therapy on the basis of therapist limit setting. He found it 'highly unlikely' that this would happen, but 'more constructive than continuing it on a false basis'.

At the difficult edge it may not be quite as unlikely. I remember a client who asked me how I preferred to have sex with my husband. This was in the context of his wish for more reciprocal disclosures of intimate experiences between us. While I accepted and empathised with his wish for reciprocity, I also told him I couldn't answer his question; it wouldn't feel right for me to do so. He then rose and said that he'd not disclose all about himself if I were not willing to do the same, and then he left, slamming the door behind him. Reflecting on the experience afterwards, I ended up thinking that he chose very wisely – I could never become the therapist he apparently wanted; never get closer to a kind of friendship relationship with him. Had I answered his question, he might have stayed, but we would surely, then, have been continuing on a false basis, as Rogers put it, and sooner or later I'd have had to apologise to him for answering a question I felt I shouldn't have answered and tell him that I'd be more careful not to do so in the future. Particularly at the difficult edge it is well to remember that even if a therapist can help most clients, they cannot help all clients.

Idiosyncratic limits

Therapist limits are, of course, not set in stone. Most of the limits that emerge in a therapy relationship are flexible, depending on the situation from moment to moment. A frequent client request is, for example, to have more time. This is a request therapists can sometimes accommodate and sometimes not, depending on their own calendar and other factors.

Nevertheless, in my therapy practice, I did have a few limits that were pretty much set in stone. To a certain degree, these limits may have been idiosyncratic, not shared by other therapists or only by a few other therapists. For example, being a relatively reserved and private person, I would probably not have responded differently from the way I described on p. 183 in any other situation where a client asked me how I had sex with my husband or something equally intimate and private.

I also had a pretty inflexible, premeditated limit about threatening and aggressive behaviour during sessions, whether towards me or towards my belongings, since I worked with some people who, the staff on their ward told me, could become very aggressive. First, I always made sure with all clients, by placing my shawl on the chair, that I would be the one nearest to the door of my office. Furthermore, it was one which I had become accustomed to sitting in – I actually concentrated less well when I did not sit in that chair. Second, I had made up my mind that I'd leave the room the minute I felt threatened by a client's aggressive behaviour. I wouldn't stop to speculate, even less to negotiate, whether my perception of threat was accurate or not, since in any case, I couldn't work properly if I felt scared and in need of immediately getting away from that scary place. I would not ask the client to behave differently, or to leave – I wouldn't have expectations of the client, with the risk of experiencing negative regard for the client if the client did not live up to my expectations. The responsibility to feel properly protected was purely my own. I would not get into a situation that might feel like asking the rain to stop raining because I was not properly dressed. Instead, I would get out of the rain to put on some protective clothes, which, in this case, would mean going to ask a staff member from the client's ward to collect him or her. I felt very secure with all clients with my plan and it turned out that I only once needed to act when, in an outburst of anger a client turned over a little lamp on the table next to him. I felt scared at this escalation of his expressions of anger and immediately rose and went to the door, whereupon the client apologised and said that nothing like this would happen again. I was satisfied with this, felt secure, sat down and we continued the session. I suspect, but can of course not know, that my firm resolution to get out of the way of what I experienced as threatening behaviour had a positive effect in this situation, and perhaps also in others, as if my sense of security in my capacity to protect myself made the threatening behaviour seem outlandish.

This limit of mine, with respect to aggressive behaviour during sessions, may also be considered idiosyncratic in the sense that it allowed for my being neither big and strong nor physically courageous – other therapist's limits in situations like the one described above may vary widely from mine. As Jin Wu wrote in the email discussion (see p. 182): 'The client-centered therapist checks with themself to see if honoring a client's request would compromise their ability to provide the conditions, so such limits vary a great deal from therapist to therapist'. And in the email discussion, Dorothy Morgan states that 'limits and limit setting would fall within the category of genuineness', implying, as Jin Wu said, that they will vary a great deal from therapist to therapist. Therefore, the examples of limits and limit setting I have offered from my own practice in this chapter are certainly not meant as recommendations for other therapists to do likewise. They are only meant to be illustrative of ways limit setting can become necessary in work at the difficult edge. We each have our own unique needs and ways of being with respect to protecting our capacity to experience unconditional positive regard and empathic understanding of the client.

Nevertheless, let me give a final example of another idiosyncratic limitation from my own working life. As I gained experience I discovered that I could not tolerate more than two depressed clients in a row. Sometimes when I happened to have three I felt 'contaminated' by the hopelessness of the previous two, and I started identifying with the hopelessness of the third about his or her prospects for the future. I ended up feeling as hopeless, or almost as hopeless, about everything as the third client did. When I noticed the possibility of that sequence occurring I rescheduled one of the clients to another day of the week.

It may be relevant to mention in this connection that I would only explain why I did this, or any other of my limit setting, if an explanation was requested by the client. I did not want to interfere from my own perspective more than absolutely necessary, and mostly clients did not request explanations. Clients ordinarily just respond with acceptance of the therapist's limits, precisely like Rogers' client did not request any explanation for his 'no' to have sexual intercourse with her and Rogers did not offer any explanation either (see p. 174).

Likewise, I did not offer a 'list' of my limits for negotiation with new clients, since I couldn't know which ones, if any, they'd challenge and they might also come to challenge a hitherto unknown limit of mine that I couldn't know of in advance. Also, demarcating various limits in the first session seemed unnecessarily rigid – if and when challenged, the limits would emerge in due time. Furthermore, most of my limits, particularly the more idiosyncratic ones, would ordinarily not be up for negotiation if they were challenged. The only 'limits' I found it necessary to agree with the client about at the end of the first session were when, where and for how long we were to meet next time – if, indeed, the client wanted a next time.

References

Barrett-Lennard, G (1998) *Carl Rogers' Helping System. Journey and substance.* London: Sage Publications.

Moon, K (2001) Nondirective client-centered therapy with children. *The Person-Centered Journal, 8*(1), 43–53.

Prouty, G (1994) *Theoretical Evolutions in Person-Centered/Experiential Therapy: Applications to schizophrenic and retarded psychoses.* Westport, CT: Praeger.

Prouty, G, Van Werde, D & Pörtner, M (2002) *Pre-Therapy: Reaching contact-impaired clients.* Ross-on-Wye: PCCS Books.

Rogers, CR (1942) *Counseling and Psychotherapy.* Boston: Houghton Mifflin.

Rogers, CR (1951) *Client-Centered Therapy.* Boston: Houghton Mifflin.

Rogers, CR (1957) The necessary and sufficient conditions of therapeutic personality change. *Journal of Consulting Psychology, 21*(2), 95–103.

Rogers, CR (1959) A theory of therapy, personality and interpersonal relationships, as developed in the client-centered framework. In S Koch (Ed) *Psychology: A study of science, Vol. 3: Formulations of the person and the social context* (pp. 184–256). New York: McGraw-Hill.

Rogers, C, Gendlin, E, Kiesler, D & Truax, C (1967) *The Therapeutic Relationship and Its Impact: A study of psychotherapy with schizophrenics.* Madison, WI: University of Wisconsin Press.

Sanders, P (2007) *The Contact Work Primer: An introduction to Pre-Therapy and the work of Garry Prouty.* Ross-on-Wye: PCCS Books.

Sommerbeck, L (2002) The Wisconsin watershed – Or the universality of CCT. *The Person-Centered Journal, 9*(2), 140–57.

Sommerbeck, L (2012) Being non-directive in directive settings. *Person-Centered & Experiential Psychotherapies, 11*(3), 173–90.

Part 3
Research that supports practice

An investigation of the effectiveness of person-centred therapy for 'psychotic' processes in adult clients 14

Wendy Traynor

Introduction

An increasing number of person-centred practitioners working in primary care, third sector charities and private practice encounter clients with what are sometimes referred to as 'psychotic' processes, involving a wide range of experiences including hearing voices, other hallucinations, delusions, dissociation, unusual thoughts, feelings and behaviour.

In person-centred therapy (PCT), severe and enduring distress was recognised as an important challenge over 50 years ago by Rogers, Gendlin, Kiesler and Truax (1967) when designing the Wisconsin schizophrenia project. Although seen by many as a disappointment (Kirschenbaum, 2007), it is increasingly obvious that this study was significant in demonstrating some degree of positive outcomes in this client group. This was especially the case when 'psychological contact' could be established with the clients (Rogers et al., 1967).

This chapter summarises my ongoing research with practitioners who work with people with psychotic processes, and their clients. I have personally struggled with the use of the word 'psychotic' but the term is used widely by both practitioners in the field and clients. I have used it in this chapter with some sense of discomfort but also struggled with alternative descriptions. When I am working with clients I focus on the person and what they bring but have found both mainstream literature associated with this description and critical stances (e.g., Read, 2004; Bentall, 2009) helpful in the work. I have often needed to communicate clearly with psychiatrists and workers in early intervention in psychosis teams when working as part of a multi-disciplinary care provision for clients, whilst keeping a person-centred stance at the heart of the work with the client. This is not an easy position and I have had concerns of colluding with a

I want to thank my supervisors, managers and my PhD supervisory team (Professor Robert Elliott and Professor Mick Cooper). The feedback from participants and clients has enabled me to continue this research and climb over the inevitable hurdles. The wider mental health community and those who support the de-pathologising of distress have also been important sources of inspiration for me.

medicalised stance and the power issues associated with this, even though many of my clients have used medical-model terminology themselves. My personal preference is to engage with a process of formulation rather than diagnosis.

A person-centred understanding of psychosis was offered by Rogers as early as 1951 in his book *Client-Centered Therapy: Its current practices, implications and theory* and later developed by a range of authors, for example, Berghofer (1996); Dekeyser, Prouty & Elliott (2007); Holdstock and Rogers (1977); Prouty (1994, 2001, 2002, 2008); Sanders (2007a, b); Shlien, (2003); Sommerbeck (2003, 2007); Van Werde (2008); Warner (2007, 2013) and most recently, Margaret Warner (this volume, Chapter 10).

Compared with psychodynamic and cognitive approaches, person-centred publications on this topic are relatively scarce and it should go without saying that further research is needed to increase understanding of how clients who hear voices, have intrusive thoughts, and unusual perceptions or ideas may experience person-centred and experiential psychotherapies. There is also the hope of gaining more understanding of whether person-centred and experiential therapies may be effective and elements of how this process occurs. Research and theoretical- and practice-related literature relating to more complex process continues to be published (see above) to support both trainees and more experienced practitioners. However, many questions remain unanswered and many myths surrounding the person-centred approach in general, and with this client group in particular, prevail.

My initial drive to conduct research began in a very limited and tentative way, with the quest for survival of the PCT modality in a fierce and critical climate of working with clients with complex processes, with an advancing tide of evidence-based practice. This drive soon shifted to embrace a deeper and more genuine curiosity and focus. Regardless of my previous preference for PCT, I wanted to develop a research agenda whose outcomes could contribute towards an understanding of optimal treatment on an individual therapy level, as well as work within multi-disciplinary teams. My aims were:

- to understand more of what really mattered for clients

- to unravel what practice elements appeared to help and which elements were less helpful or hindering

- to identify the changes which may occur

- to develop further understanding of what might constitute best practice in complex process work

- to understand how elements of good practice might be fine-tuned

- to determine what sort of changes might occur which may be partly or wholly attributed to the therapy

- to identify wider contextual issues which might impact on client experiences and outcomes

- to identify possible emerging contra-indications or negative experiences.

My research

I set out to discover whether person-centred and experiential therapies are effective for clients who have unusual experiences or 'psychotic processes' in three related studies. The first involved interviewing 20 practitioners, the second involved interviewing 20 adult clients and the third study, ongoing at the time of writing, consists of a Hermeneutic Single Case Efficacy Design (HSCED) (Elliott, 2001, 2002). I had to change my initial research design after I was granted National Health Service (NHS) ethical approval for an open clinical trial (OCT) but recruitment was difficult due to changes in National Institute for Health and Care Excellence (NICE) guidelines (National Collaborating Centre for Mental Health (NCCMH)/ NICE, 2003) – that cognitive behavioural therapy (CBT) should be the first line of treatment. This resulted in sites and individuals dropping out of my study, as they struggled to retain contracts and keep services open in a difficult economic climate where research was not the immediate priority. I modified my design to replace my planned OCT with a study in which I directly asked clients about their experiences of therapy and this received ethical approval by both the University of Strathclyde and the NHS. The HSCED data were generated for my final study by using outcome measures throughout therapy with a client with psychotic process. The Change Interview was administered by a team of researchers who were not offering therapy to the participant clients, generating both qualitative and quantitative data. At the time of writing, this final study is in the process of data analysis.[1]

The studies are concerned with PCT as a mode of practice which focuses more on, and encapsulates, 'ways of being' rather than 'techniques' in the context of unusual experiences and complex process. The approach has often been the source of critical scrutiny although many of the elements of the PCT approach such as empathy and power dynamics are consistently cited in survivor literature. Critiques which question the PCT stance as benign at best or, at worst, dangerous, have struggled to evidence their view and Sommerbeck (2003) refuted such critiques with case examples. In the meantime I, along with other person-centred therapists working in this field, sought supplementary training in additional approaches in the context of a climate of evidence-based practice required by NICE (NCCMH/ NICE, 2003; NICE 2004). This led many to adopt a more pluralistic stance with the person-centred model at the heart of their practice and values.

Private communications, conference presentations, anecdotal accounts and my own practice over a period of twenty years are replete with many examples of successful therapeutic work in this area of client experience, and I embarked

---

1. All names of participating clients and practitioners have been changed to maintain confidentility.

on this doctoral research study whilst continuing to work as a therapist. I often encountered other therapists in a similar position – facing complexity in the therapy room at the same time as having to face the wider challenge of the professional political context. PCT practitioners have to give a good account of why they are offering a comparatively less-researched approach than, for example, cognitive behavioural approaches, with the medical model and associated diagnostic framework in the background.

Since working in a fundamentally person-centred way could be so easily challenged, my research began by focusing on unpicking existing research, and listening to the stories of clients, practitioners and significant others. I conducted the research whilst continuing to negotiate a world in which there was considerable lack of understanding and trust between therapists of different models. I became determined to build bridges, understand and communicate with professionals working with this client group whilst always keeping the client and their experiences at the centre of the work.

Study 1

My first study involved interviewing 20 practitioners who had worked with a minimum of one client who had heard voices, hallucinated, had paranoid ideas, delusions or other unusual experiences which the medical model may refer to as psychotic experiences. After ethical approval, participant practitioners[2] were recruited from notices in counselling journals, person-centred websites, organisations and groups, and by word of mouth.

I conducted unstructured interviews with prompts focusing on the following key areas:

- training, background and work context
- experience of working with clients in 'psychotic' process
- the practice offered to such clients, including any difference from usual practice
- specific aspects of practice which seemed particularly helpful to clients.

The latter part of the interviews focused on:

- perceived changes in clients and how the participants came to this view (e.g., evaluation tools, observations or client feedback)
- unhelpful practice and any possible negative outcomes
- additional issues which they felt were important.

2. Participant 'practitioners' comprised a range of qualified helping professionals including counsellors, psychotherapists and psychologists. They are referred to generically as 'practitioners' throughout the summary of results.

Fifteen interviews were conducted face to face and five were by telephone. Debriefing was offered as needed.

The practitioners discussed over 40 clients in total. The data are presented with a focus on *episodes of therapy* rather than on the practitioner, as practice often developed over time so later practice with clients was different from earlier practice and there was obvious variation in data for each client episode. Furthermore, since most practitioners described more than one client, their practice often changed over time as they accessed further post-qualification training or resources, for example, Pre-Therapy. Therefore practitioners showed how they increased in experience and skills and went on to demonstrate this in sessions with clients. Themes in results are therefore also more accurately captured by reporting incidents rather than numbers of practitioners.

The data were analysed and audited using the principles of grounded theory (Glaser & Strauss, 1967, as interpreted by Rennie, Phillips & Quartaro, 1988) allowing themes to emerge from the data. The results were then grouped into categories and subcategories as themes recurred.

Study 1 outcomes

3 (out of 20) practitioners simply used the core person-centred approach for *all* clients including those clients who were experiencing 'psychotic processes'.

17 (out of 20) practitioners had developed their practice after training and reading and worked differently from a classical model – particularly incorporating Pre-Therapy and contact reflections (Prouty et al., 2002) (11 practitioners).[3] Each practitioner discussed one or more clients and so different iterations of person-centred practice, including developments such as Pre-Therapy, may have been experienced by clients who were seen later on a practice timeline in a practitioner's career.

- **6 practitioners** described general ways in which they tried to make contact with clients such as observing and gently feeding back an invitation for contact whilst another described verbally checking out if clients were in contact with them. Other practitioners mentioned very specific practices which they had developed and found useful with this type of complex client process.

- **11 practitioners** sometimes used Pre-Therapy as a way of working and all 11 found this effective with clients. Some practitioners found Pre-Therapy to be a revelation and worked with improved confidence, seeing outcomes such as increased links to reality. Some practitioners had attended short courses in Pre-Therapy which had impacted on their practice and others described working closely to 'Garry's book' (Prouty, et al., 2002).

---

3. For a review of Pre-Therapy research see Chapter 15 by Dekeyser, Prouty and Elliott.

> ▷ *1 practitioner* said, 'The Garry Prouty reflections were useful in trying to establish a connection between both of us – working in the here and now and reinforcing the reality of the moment.'

> ▷ *1 practitioner* described using contact reflections in the context of an acute ward with one client over a number of occasions. She described how a member of the nursing staff said, 'Why are you talking to him, you won't get any sense out of him!' At first the client was seemingly unresponsive and was sometimes 'taking to aliens that he saw' but then suddenly started to talk to the practitioner and showed her drawings in between periods of being less in contact. Over time he became more interested in engaging with the practitioner and they explored the feelings beneath some of the unusual content of his experiences.

- Other specific practices informed by specific theory were also mentioned.

  > ▷ The value of Margaret Warner's work (2001) in difficult client processes was acknowledged (4 practitioners). One practitioner specifically followed her 'fragile process' suggestions with a client, staying close to the client's words.

Specific themes

Various elements of building a person-centred therapeutic (PCT) relationship and therapeutic conditions were described as important:

- **Genuine care (8 practitioners)** e.g., showing warmth, compassion and love

- **Relational depth (7 practitioners)**
  > ▷ *1 practitioner* said that there were 'those moments where you meet eye-to-eye and something happens … special moments … soul moments … as if a barrier has gone – a spiritual connection.'
  > ▷ *1 practitioner* described the relationship as empowered and deep.
  > ▷ However the research also showed examples of how some vulnerable clients could not cope with relational depth and need space and less intensity to feel safe and maintain contact.

- **Importance of being real, striving to be real, or use of self (6 practitioners)**
  > ▷ *1 practitioner* commented that 'the relationship is the therapy' – especially important where people have been stigmatised in relation to mental health issues.

- **Minimising the power dynamic and maximising empowerment (6 practitioners)**

- **Unconditional positive regard (UPR) (15 practitioners).** Themes included accepting all parts of the client.

  ▷ *1 practitioner* commented that UPR is crucial for clients who experience psychotic process as they often feel guilt, shame or rejection.

  ▷ *1 practitioner* commented, 'I think that acceptance is a big thing. If you accept someone as they are they can show more of themselves – and become more confident in themselves as well, and then begin to reflect themselves on whether they want to change.' They went on to explain that clients who have often had little power can feel empowered by such acceptance and develop courage to take power back.

- **Taking care in the use of congruence (8 practitioners).** Congruence clearly required particular consideration with some variation in approach.

  ▷ *2 practitioners* felt that clients in psychotic process could be more sensitive to incongruence and that it was important to be congruent.

  ▷ *2 practitioners* felt that less congruence was appropriate and that there needed to be less edge-of-awareness work or more negotiating with sensitive or fragile clients regarding what was safe to 'name'.

  ▷ *4 practitioners* were particularly sensitive in their use of congruence and they varied their approach according to perceived individual client needs and processes.

- **Empathy, emphasising the need for deep empathy and staying close to clients (8 practitioners)**

Specific strategies

Working with 'psychotic content':

- **Ways of working with the clients' voices, hallucinations, unusual ideas (14 practitioners)**

  ▷ *3 practitioners* discussed simply entering into the client's reality or accepting the client's reality, e.g., staying with a client's world.

  ▷ *3 practitioners* described staying with 'the client's frame' and owning their own, different reality from the client.

  ▷ *3 practitioners* discussed staying in the client's frame whilst privately holding their own sense of what was 'not true to them'.

  ▷ *5 practitioners* sometimes felt distracted when holding two realities. For example, one practitioner reflected that she had no idea what was true, and it was not her job to judge. She tried to put aside her awareness of the potential difference between her reality and the client's, and just try to understand what her client believed.

- **Dealing with the practitioners' own reactions to hearing voices, hallucinations or psychotic content of sessions (5 practitioners)**

  ▷ Some initially felt fear, shock or unsettled and tried to avoid distraction or panic. However, over time they described growing increasingly comfortable with such material, often processing it in supervision. Having a supervisor with a mental health background was helpful. One practitioner commented, 'I felt so challenged by this client. Could I be with her? It was a real test of my beliefs in the person-centred approach. Will it be enough? Will I be enough?' She went on to explain how she attempted to meet her client where she was and stay close to her process. Increasing familiarity with 'psychotic material' can enable the practitioner 'to stay with' the client.

  ▷ Self-care in order to stay with the client and deal with sometimes 'horrific' material, describing a need to ground themselves in, and after, sessions.

  ▷ The need to adapt parameters to accommodate client needs (8 practitioners with 20 responses[4] on this theme)

  ▷ The use of space (4 responses) e.g., working in a large space was necessary for some clients whilst respecting the distance and closeness needed by specific clients as needs changed.

  ▷ Attention to boundaries and contracting, including the need for flexibility regarding client telephone calls, missed sessions or the length of sessions. Practitioners also described the importance of having a contract the client understood and having firm boundaries which were not rigid.

Other specific strategies

- **Supporting the coping strategies or educational elements offered to the client by other practitioners within the multi-disciplinary context of care (6 practitioners).** Some practitioners supported clients to understand what was happening to them but avoided giving actual advice.

- **Getting beyond labels and focusing on the person rather than the 'illness' or diagnosis (10 practitioners)**

  ▷ *1 practitioner* commented, 'Six months into the counselling Emma told me that she had bad news for me. The doctor had told her that she had schizophrenia and depression. I asked her what this meant to her. 'I am a maniac,' Emma said. The practitioner responded by saying, 'I see and hear how upset you are, devastated by this news. You are Emma to me. I feel very close to you right now.' She explained that she valued Emma. She described how Emma became more trusting of her and opened up issues in a deep counselling relationship.

---

4. A single participant practitioner or client might make several responses, so the number of responses will not tally with either the number of practitioners or clients who responded.

> ▷ *1 practitioner* said, 'If you want me to identify the active ingredient … it was being non-labelling, not making assumptions, taking each moment afresh and trying to understand [clients as people].'

- **Exercising particular care and attention with such complex client processes (15 responses).** Several practitioners wanted or needed more than one practitioner in the room or to have co-practitioners.

  > ▷ *1 practitioner* explained that this was to hold the process and for practitioners to be able to look after each other if a situation was demanding.

- **Using a multi-disciplinary approach for vulnerable clients and to help the practitioner to stay with the client (7 practitioners)**

- **Supporting the client to manage risks to self and others (6 practitioners)**

Perceived changes in clients

30 (out of 40) clients were described by their practitioners as more connected

- **Increased contact with reality being achieved (9 practitioners)**

  > ▷ *1 practitioner* explained that she and the client began to have intermittent contact where they would share that reality for a few moments or a few minutes.

  > ▷ *1 practitioner* described 'seeing someone, for want of a better word, come out of a psychosis, become more connected within a relationship and less distressed.'

  > ▷ *24 responses* related to outcomes associated specifically with improved social skills and ability to be with and relate to others. This was the most frequently mentioned outcome. Socialising was described as being easier for many clients discussed. One client, described as initially going for days without saying anything other than 'hello' to anybody moved to 'striking up conversations with people and … striking up almost friendships'. A further example described a 'disconnected' person becoming able to attend an occupational therapy group and engage in activities.

- **Decreased difficulties with problematic experiences (31 responses)**

  > ▷ *2 practitioners* reported clients having less need for treatment. One client was able to withdraw from antipsychotic medication.

  > ▷ *4 practitioners* identified the client's improved ability to manage voices or hallucinations. Typical comments referred to clients accepting their voices, learning to cope more effectively with voices or other hallucinations, and becoming less likely to act upon them.

▷ *1 client* recognised alcohol as a trigger to worsen hallucinations and consequently stopped drinking.

▷ *2 responses* referred to a reduction in voices or hallucinations whilst one client reported to their practitioner that the voices became quieter.

▷ *4 practitioners* described clients being more accepting of hallucinations.

▷ *10 responses* described improvement in mood/anxiety levels. One practitioner saw the mood lift in all three of their clients.

▷ *9 responses* recorded reduced risk of harm to self or others, e.g., one client, who previously discussed delusional beliefs regarding his family, felt that the sessions helped him to process feelings such as anger and hatred and felt fewer urges to hurt others.

- **Improvements in sense of self (24 responses)**

  ▷ *3 practitioners* reported that their clients said they felt more accepted/less judged and a further three clients were described as showing an increase in self-acceptance/confidence and in one example the client became more accepting of others.

  ▷ *6 clients* felt more in control/empowered.

  ▷ *7 clients* showed an increase in insight or self-awareness

  ▷ *5 clients* were more integrated. Three responses involved clients who explored issues around sexual identity with one moving from confusion to entering a relationship at the end of therapy.

- **Improvements in quality of life (15 responses)**

  ▷ *9 clients* had increased resilience and were more able to cope with life and stressful situations

  ▷ *6 practitioners* reported general improvements in their clients.

Negative responses or contra-indications (responses from 3 practitioners)

- Practitioners discussed the need for tempering of intensity, identifying potential triggers if applicable and being provided with adequate guidance. Some clients might be identified as being better suited to other types of therapy and could be referred if appropriate.

Study 2

This study comprised interviews with 20 clients who had experiences of hearing voices, hallucinations, paranoia, unusual ideas or psychotic experiences and had received person-centred or experiential therapy. Following ethical approval for the study and a recruitment phase, the participant clients[5] were interviewed

---

5. Participant clients are referred to as 'clients' in the following results.

using The Change Interview (Elliott et al., 2001) including a semi-structured schedule with scales focusing on the experience of therapy, helpful and less helpful experiences of therapy, changes perceived by the clients and other contextual issues. The questions prompted discussion about what changes may be attributed to the therapy and other potentially impacting factors. The aim was to compare the client data with the practitioner data and determine if there were key overlaps or differences in themes relating to helpful or less helpful practices, therapy experiences and perceived changes.

At the time of writing the data analysis is incomplete. A preliminary analysis of the change section of the set interviews charts where clients have listed and scored changes. Clients also rated on a scale whether the change was important, whether the change may have occurred without the therapy and how surprising the changes were. The data were then cross-analysed to the emerging themes developed from grounded theory analysis, along with some rich case examples. Data analysis already shows some important points for consideration in practice and a selection is presented here.

Study 2 outcomes

Emerging themes in helpful and less helpful practitioner practices, plus perceived changes and discussions of outcomes

The first 15 client interviews resulted in a total of 97 reported changes which clients felt were partly or totally due to the therapy. Forty-six of these changes were graded by clients on the change charts (some clients discussed changes in other ways without scoring them) and 80% (37 out of 46) charted changes which they felt were unlikely/very unlikely to have occurred without the therapy.

- **6 (out of 15) clients listed changes in voices/unusual experiences**
  Examples included feeling that things were more real.
    - ▷ *1 client* described increased reflection regarding voices and greater sense of reality.
    - ▷ *1 client* stated that 'very scary stuff' in their peripheral vision went away.
    - ▷ *2 clients* said that voices became less intense and less frequent and in one case less problematic.
    - ▷ *1 client* stated that they experienced fewer unusual thoughts.

The client participants did not necessarily find their voices or unusual experiences problematic or want to focus on them in the therapy. Even if they were troublesome, clients sometimes focused on the underlying issues and did not tell the practitioner about the voices or unusual experiences for a variety of reasons, including because the experiences did not seem relevant to the client.

Some clients found reduction in such unusual experiences, even if not discussed with the practitioner.

- **Normalising unusual experiences (5 clients)**
  - ▷ Clients described feeling less weird, less different, less 'mad' and more self-accepting and accepting of their voices. The need to normalise unusual experiences was mentioned as well as the need to focus on *what a person can do* instead of *what is wrong*.

- **Positive changes in mood and anxiety (4 clients).** Examples of changes in anxiety included improved coping with anxiety, feeling less agitated and easier to relax.
  - ▷ *1 client* said that they no longer experienced panic attacks.
  - ▷ *3 clients* said that they felt less depressed.
  - ▷ *1 client* had previously felt so low that they were off work but experienced enormous positive change.
  - ▷ *4 clients* noticed a change in their anger and described changes such as feeling less anger, less build-up of anger and being more in control of emotions.

- **Increased general activity (2 clients).** Positive changes in thinking and behaviour (8 clients), including the less frequent occurrence of obsessive compulsive behaviours.
  - ▷ *1 client* had stopped washing in bleach and moved on to feel less contaminated and dirty.
  - ▷ *6 clients* discussed positive shifts in perspective whilst others spoke of increased hope or insight.

- **Improvements in suicidal ideation/risk (3 clients)**
  - ▷ *2 clients* said that they became less suicidal.
  - ▷ *1 client* said that the therapy kept them alive.

- **Improvements in social functioning (24 responses)**
  - ▷ *3 clients* saw improvements in intimate relationships or their abilities to make healthier judgements about these.
  - ▷ *6 clients* noted improvements in general relationships with friends, family and others and discussed examples such as being more able to make friends and to go out and mix socially. Three other clients stated that they became more assertive with others.
  - ▷ *12 clients* mentioned changes in social skills and gave examples such as being more able to keep appropriate boundaries, becoming more expressive, more humble, more able to apologise and becoming more accepting of others.

- **Better coping (3 clients)**
    - ▷ *3 clients* described improvements in coping as the therapy progressed.
    - ▷ *1 client* felt more able to cope with grief.
    - ▷ *2 clients* felt more able to access education.
- **Changes in self (33 responses)** including clients feeling more self-value, a stronger sense of self, more self-respect and more connected to self.
    - ▷ *1 client* said, 'I know myself better' whilst another said, 'I became fully me – I'd never been me'.
    - ▷ *Other clients* described becoming more aware of their needs and emotions.

Cross-analysis

The cross-analysis of emerging qualitative data highlighted practice considerations. Clients often highlighted a person-centred ethos in their comments. Comments relating to helpful practice included:

- a flexible approach
- being heard by a practitioner who was real and present
- being supported to work at their own pace and not to be pushed to discuss issues unless they felt ready
- painful exploration could be very helpful if not initiated under pressure.

Clients also identified the following unhelpful practitioner attributes:

- unwelcome directivity
- exaggerating emotions too much
- being judged
- practitioner not being active in the relationship.

Conclusions

Practitioner data and client data show similarities in both important and helpful practice and outcomes. Clients and practitioners both placed great importance on the normalisation of experiences and getting beyond labels. This reflects the person-centred theoretical position regarding language, labels and diagnosis. The person-centred ethos stood out in the qualities which were perceived by both groups as important for, and helpful to, therapy. Experiences identified that were not helpful – such as unwanted therapist directivity – were those that generally did not fit with a person-centred stance.

The majority of clients in both studies showed significant improvement in many areas including sense of self, identity, social functioning, and frequency and distress caused by unusual experiences (including voice-hearing). In short, the most troubling symptoms of a medical model of diagnosis of 'psychosis' were reported as improved. In addition, when working with person-centred practitioners, clients were able to describe how stigmatisation and social pressure affected their comfort regarding disclosure of symptoms. Furthermore, some explained that they did not necessarily experience their symptoms as disturbing, and the non-judgemental attitude of the practitioner allowed them to discuss this.

Both clients and practitioners repeatedly gave examples of working with symbolic meaning, emotional content or underlying issues rather than symptoms or diagnosis unless the latter was led by the client.

Regarding further training and professional development, the most popular additional practice was Pre-Therapy. The introduction of Pre-Therapy or contact work to therapeutic practice or within the context of a supportive relationship was seen to increase the ability of practitioners to make contact with clients and increase the likelihood of a positive therapeutic relationship. The work of Margaret Warner (2000, 2001, 2002, 2007) was also a strong influence for several practitioners. In PCT allied with Pre-Therapy the task of psychotherapy is to help the person achieve, through a special relationship with the practitioner, good communication within themselves. Once this is achieved the client can communicate more freely and more effectively with others (Rogers, 1961, p. 330).

Paralleling Warner (2001) and Mearns (2003), the results suggest that responsible practice when working with psychotic processes may involve sensitive and appropriate adjustment of the therapeutic setting. Supervision and careful reflection were seen to be important to enable practitioners to discern if and when boundaries should be extended or tightened. For example, some clients may feel safer or more comfortable working in larger spaces than a standard therapy room, whilst other clients might want to lie on the floor on cushions with the practitioner sitting on a cushion at the same level.

In contrast, in some instances it may be important for the practitioner to keep very clear and explicit time boundaries, have clear risk-management contingencies and carefully observe the limits of their competence, for example, considering referring if the client may need a higher level of care. This can help to reduce the risk of practitioner burn-out and supports client safety and continuity of care.

The most dramatic and general finding in this study is the role of PCT in enhancing client social and interpersonal skills. Given the degree of social isolation and interpersonal avoidance in this population, this kind of change is essential for helping clients improve their quality of life (Davidson & Staynor, 1997/1999; Harding, 1987). This is consistent with the results of the Wisconsin project (Rogers, 1967) and the Essen study (Teusch, 1990).

There is no doubt that this work can be demanding and unsettling for practitioners, particularly when the practitioner is inexperienced. While this type of work is not for everyone, the data show that experience and support often help practitioners to stay grounded and in turn enable them to support clients through positive change.

This research is aimed at improving the care and ultimate wellbeing of this underserved and often disadvantaged client group. Clearly more research is needed in this area and the present studies might inspire others to conduct research on person-centred therapy with this client group. The results so far are encouraging.

References

Bentall, RP (2009) *Doctoring the Mind: Why psychiatric treatments fail*. London: Allen Lane.

Berghofer, G (1996) Dealing with schizophrenia: A person-centered approach providing care to long-term patients in a supported residential service in Vienna. In R Hutterer, G Pawlowsky, PF Schmid & R Stipsits (Eds) *Client-Centered and Experiential Psychotherapy: A paradigm in motion* (pp. 481–94). Frankfurt am Main: Peter Lang.

Davidson, L & Stayner, D (1997) Loss, loneliness, and the desire for love: Perspectives on the social lives of people with schizophrenia. *Psychiatric Rehabilitation Journal, 20*, 3–12. Reprinted (1999) in RP Marinelli & AE Dell Orto (Eds) *The Psychological and Social Impact of Disability* (4th ed) (pp. 220–35). New York: Springer.

Dekeyser, M, Prouty, G & Elliott, R (2007) Pre-Therapy process and outcome: A review of research instruments and findings. *Person-Centered & Experiential Psychotherapies, 7*, 37–55.

Elliott, R (2001) Hermeneutic single case efficacy design (HSCED): An overview. In KJ Schneider, JFT Bugental & JF Fraser (Eds) *Handbook of Humanistic Psychology* (pp. 315–24). Thousand Oaks, CA: Sage.

Elliott, R (2002) Hermaneutic single case efficacy design. *Psychotherapy Research, 12*, 1–21.

Elliott, R, Slatick, E & Urman, M (2001) Qualitative change process research on psychotherapy: Alternative strategies. In J Frommer & D Rennie (Eds) *Qualitative Psychotherapy Research: Methods and methodology* (pp. 69–111). Lengerich, Germany: Pabst Science Publishers.

Glaser, BG & Strauss, AL (1967) *The Discovery of Grounded Theory: Strategies for qualitative research*. Chicago: Aldine Publishing Company.

Harding, C (1987) The Vermont longitudinal study of persons with mental illness I. *American Journal of Psychiatry, 144*, 718–26.

Holdstock, TL & Rogers, CR (1977) Person-centered theory. In RJ Corsini (Ed) *Current Personality Theories* (pp. 125–51). Itasca, IL: Peacock.

Kirschenbaum, H (2007) *The Life and Work of Carl Rogers*. Ross-on-Wye: PCCS Books.

Mearns, D (2003) What is involved in offering wider contracts to clients? In *Developing Person-Centred Counselling* (pp. 10–12). London: Sage.

National Collaborating Centre for Mental Health (NCCMH) (commissioned by the National Institute for Clinical Excellence) (2003) *Schizophrenia: Full national clinical guideline on core interventions in primary and secondary care* (pp. 90–102). London: Gaskell and the British Psychological Society.

National Institute for Health and Care Excellence (NICE) (2014) *Psychosis and Schizophrenia in Adults: Treatment and management.* Issued February 2014, last modified March 2014, NICE Clinical Guideline 178 (pp. 22–6). Retrieved 2 June 2014 from http://guidance.nice.org.uk/cg178

Prouty, G (1994) *Theoretical Evolutions in Person-Centered/Experiential Therapy. Applications to schizophrenic and retarded psychoses.* New York: Praeger.

Prouty, G (2001) Unconditional positive regard and Pre-Therapy: An exploration. In JD Bozarth & P Wilkins (Eds) *Rogers' Therapeutic Conditions: Evolution, theory and practice. Vol 3: Unconditional Positive Regard* (pp. 76–87). Ross-on Wye: PCCS Books.

Prouty, G (2002) Humanistic psychotherapy for people with schizophrenia, In D Cain & J Seeman (Eds) *Humanistic Psychotherapies: Handbook of Research and Practice* (pp. 579–601). Washington, DC: American Psychological Association.

Prouty, G (Ed) (2008) *Emerging Developments in Pre-Therapy: A Pre-Therapy reader.* Ross-on-Wye: PCCS Books.

Prouty, G, Van Werde, D & Pörtner, M (2002) *Pre-Therapy: Reaching contact-impaired clients.* Ross-on-Wye: PCCS Books.

Read, J (2004) Does 'schizophrenia' exist? Reliability and validity. In J Read, LR Mosher & RP Bentall (Eds) *Models of Madness* (pp. 43–56). Hove: Brunner-Routledge.

Rennie, D, Phillips, JR & Quartaro, GK (1988) Grounded theory: A promising approach to conceptualization in psychology? *Canadian Psychology, 29,* 139–50.

Rogers, CR (1951) *Client-Centered Therapy: Its current practices, implications and theory.* London: Constable.

Rogers, CR (1961) *On Becoming a Person: A therapist's view of psychotherapy.* London: Constable.

Rogers, CR (1967) The findings in brief. In CR Rogers, ET Gendlin, DJ Kiesler & CB Truax (Eds) *The Therapeutic Relationship and Its Impact: A study of psychotherapy with schizophrenics* (pp. 73–94). Madison, WI: University of Wisconsin Press.

Rogers, CR, Gendlin, ET, Kiesler, DJ & Truax, CB (1967) *The Therapeutic Relationship and Its Impact: A study of psychotherapy with schizophrenics.* Madison, WI: University of Wisconsin Press.

Sanders, P (Ed) (2007a) *The Contact Work Primer.* Ross-on-Wye: PCCS Books.

Sanders, P (2007b) Schizophrenia is not an illness – A response to van Blarikom. *Person-Centered & Experiential Psychotherapies, 6,* 112–28.

Shlien, JM (2003) *To Lead an Honorable Life: Invitations to think about client-centered therapy and the person-centered approach.* Ross-on-Wye: PCCS Books.

Sommerbeck, L (2003) *The Client-Centred Therapist in Psychiatric Contexts: A therapists' guide to the psychiatric landscape and its inhabitants.* Ross-on-Wye: PCCS Books.

Sommerbeck, L (2005) An evaluation of research, concepts and experiences pertaining to the universality of CCT and its application in psychiatric settings. In S Joseph & R Worsley (Eds) *Person-Centred Psychopathology: A positive psychology of mental health* (pp. 317–36). Ross-on-Wye: PCCS Books.

Teusch, L (1990) Positive effects and limitations of client-centered therapy with schizophrenic patients. In G Lietaer, J Rombauts, & R Van Balen (Eds) *Client-Centered and Experiential Psychotherapy in the Nineties* (pp. 637–44). Leuven, Belgium: Leuven University Press.

Traynor, W, Elliott, R & Cooper, M (2011) Helpful factors and outcomes in person-centered therapy with clients who experience psychotic processes: Therapists' perspectives. *Person-Centered & Experiential Psychotherapies, 10,* 89–104.

Van Werde, D (2008) The falling man: Pre-Therapy applied to somatic hallucinating. In G Prouty (Ed) *Emerging Developments in Pre-Therapy: A Pre-Therapy reader* (pp. 39–46). Ross-on-Wye: PCCS Books.

Warner, MS (2000) Person-centred therapy at the difficult edge: A developmentally based model of fragile and dissociated process. In D Mearns & B Thorne (Eds) *Person-Centred Therapy Today: New frontiers in theory and practice* (pp. 144–71). London: Sage.

Warner, MS (2001) Empathy, relational depth and difficult client process. In S Haugh & T Merry (Eds) *Rogers' Therapeutic Conditions: Evolution, theory and practice. Vol 2: Empathy* (pp. 181–91). Ross-on-Wye: PCCS Books.

Warner, MS (2002) Luke's dilemmas: A client-centered/experiential model of processing with a schizophrenic thought disorder. In JC Watson, RN Goldman & MS Warner (Eds) *Client-Centered and Experiential Psychotherapy in the 21st Century: Advances in theory, research and practice* (pp. 459–72). Ross-on-Wye: PCCS Books.

Warner, MS (2007) Client incongruence and psychopathology. In M Cooper, M O'Hara, PF Schmid, & G Wyatt (Eds) *The Handbook of Person-Centred Psychotherapy and Counselling* (pp. 154–67). Basingstoke: Palgrave Macmillan.

Warner, MS (2013) Difficult client process. In M Cooper, M O'Hara, PF Schmid & AC Bohart (Eds) *The Handbook of Person-Centred Psychotherapy and Counselling* (2nd ed) (pp. 343–58). Basingstoke: Palgrave Macmillan.

Warner, MS (2014) Client processes at the difficult edge. In P Pearce & L Sommerbeck (Eds) *Person-Centred Practice at the Difficult Edge* (pp. 121–137). Ross-on-Wye: PCCS Books.

Pre-Therapy process and outcome: A review of research instruments and findings

Mathias Dekeyser, Garry Prouty and Robert Elliott

Introduction

Pre-Therapy is a client-centred treatment to prepare psychotic persons, often with profound intellectual limitations, for regular psychotherapy (Prouty, 1994; Prouty, Van Werde & Pörtner, 1998/2002). Elements of Pre-Therapy have also been applied to other populations; for example persons with a pervasive developmental disorder (Peters, 1999; Pörtner, 1996/2000), or dementia (Van Werde & Morton, 1999; Dodds, Morton & Prouty, 2004). The theory of Pre-Therapy evolved from Rogers' suggestion that psychological contact is the first condition of a therapeutic relationship. Rogers (1957) described psychological contact in the following manner: 'All that is intended by this first condition is to specify that two people are to some degree in contact, that each makes some perceived difference in the experiential field of the other' (p. 96). Rogers scarcely explained or elaborated this concept. Even though the term clearly denotes intersubjectivity, there is considerable confusion about its scope (Sanders & Wyatt, 2002).

Psychological contact and contact functions

Prouty (1994) was the first to fill this theoretical gap (Sanders & Wyatt, 2002) by introducing two important ideas born from his clinical work. First, whereas Rogers' focus was on interaction between persons, Prouty began to systematically focus on awareness within persons. Psychological contact in the sense used by Prouty does not necessarily require two individuals. Psychological contact may also involve interaction with objects, feelings, etc. (Prouty, 1994). Second, Prouty has proposed three domains of psychological contact: reality, affect, and communication, each marked by its related *contact function*. Reality contact is awareness of people, places, things, and events. Affective contact is awareness of distinct moods, feelings, and emotions. Communicative contact is

Originally published in *Person-Centered & Experiential Psychotherapies*, 7(2), 37–55. © The World Association for Person-Centered and Experiential Psychotherapy and Counseling (WAPCEPC), reprinted by permission of Taylor & Francis Ltd, www.tandfonline.com on behalf of WAPCEPC.

the symbolisation of reality contact and affective contact to others. Therefore, in Prouty's terms, psychological contact as defined by Rogers is reconceptualised as two persons in a simultaneous and mutual reality contact. Communicative contact is an overt response that is dependent on the occurrence of other contact functions (either reality or affective). Although Prouty's work is well known within the broader field of client-centred counselling and psychotherapy, Rogers' original conceptualisation is still prevalent. This is evident in Wyatt and Sanders (2002), who presented a collection of current views on psychological contact in which most authors presented a framework of dyadic intersubjectivity, elaborated with some elements of Pre-Therapy.

Contact reflections

Various studies of psychotherapy have demonstrated relationships between therapist in-session behaviour and client processes (Hill & Lambert, 2003). In Pre-Therapy, therapists employ *contact reflections* to stimulate clients' contact functions (Prouty, 1994; Prouty et al., 2002). Contact reflections are, in the language of Buber (1964), a pointing at the concrete. They are highly literal and duplicative reflections of the client's verbal and sub-verbal process. Thus, they meet the client at their own level of expression and experiencing (Prouty, 1994; Peters, 2005). There are five basic types of contact reflection: (1) *Situational Reflections*, for example, 'Mary is sitting on the floor'; (2) *Facial Reflections*, e.g., 'You look sad', or more concretely 'There are tears in your eyes'; (3) *Word-for-Word Reflections*, as when a therapist responds to a client saying, 'The (unintelligible) is moving around the (unintelligible)', by reflecting the intelligible words or sentences; (4) *Body Reflections,* e.g., 'Your arm is in the air', or, more concretely, the therapist reflecting by putting his or her own arm in the same position; and (5) *Reiterative Reflections*, that is, repetitions of any contact reflection that has affected client expression or experiencing.

Peters (2005) has provided a viable explanation for the efficacy of contact reflections. Infants are born with a propensity to discriminate and respond to stimuli that are similar to contact reflections (Fonagy, Gergely, Jurist & Target, 2002). This propensity exists from birth and persists throughout life, to some extent even in those who are later diagnosed with an autistic disorder (Beadle-Brown & Whiten, 2004). This partially intact but persistent propensity may explain why children and adults with impaired contact functions remain sensitive to contact reflections.

Pre-Therapy research

Many practitioners find Pre-Therapy a powerful method for working with contact-impaired clients. Caregivers who begin to integrate elements of Pre-Therapy in their work experience a decrease of behaviour problems in their patients (Ondracek, 2004). Over the last thirty years, a handful of independent studies have provided preliminary evidence that supports these clinical reports. As far as we know, these are the only studies of psychological contact to date and there is a clear need for more research on theories of psychological contact and their applications (Sanders & Wyatt, 2002). In support of future studies, we present a thorough review of Pre-Therapy research instruments and findings. We present: (1) an overview of instruments that have been used in Pre-Therapy studies; (2) a review of their validity; and (3) reliability; and (4) a summary of Pre-Therapy outcome findings.

Measures of contact

From the start, Pre-Therapy researchers have measured contact functions by observing clients' behaviour in interaction with others. The term *contact behaviour* refers to communication that demonstrates psychological contact (Prouty, 1994). Pre-Therapy researchers thus screen clients' verbal and non-verbal expressions for markers of contact, alternatively conceived of as *client contact responses* (Hinterkopf, Prouty & Brunswick, 1979; Prouty, 1990) or *communicative signs* (Dinacci, 1997). Occasionally, researchers have tried to observe the use of *contact reflections*. Four known measures of client contact behaviour presently exist.

The Pre-Therapy Rating Scale

Hinterkopf et al. (1979) developed the first version of the Pre-Therapy Rating Scale (PTRS-1) to assess client contact behaviour in semi-structured interviews. The interviewer follows the Pre-Therapy Questionnaire, asking items such as: 'What did you have for lunch today?' or 'How do you feel about the doctor on your ward?' Raters observe the interview twice, once from behind a one-way screen and then a second time on videotape. One scoring unit is a client's complete response to one question in the interview. Each response is rated on four categories: (1) Communication of Basic Reality; (2) Emotive Words; (3) Emotive Words with Corresponding Affect; and (4) Failure to Communicate Basic Reality and Affect. Each category is defined by a set of markers and the score for that category is the number of responses containing at least one marker. For example, an explicit reference to a concrete person is a marker for Communication of Basic Reality. If this marker is detected in a response, the observer adds one to Communication of Basic Reality. The maximum score for each category is the number of questions in the interview. The PTRS-1 does not provide a total score. Many of the contact markers defined in the PTRS-1 were later used by Prouty (1990) to develop a second version of the PTRS (PTRS-2) (De Vre, 1992). The contact response categories in this scale are: (1) Reality defined as references to people, places, things, and events; (2) Affect defined as the symbolisation of feelings, moods, and emotions; (3) Social Communication defined as the use of meaningful language; and (4) Psychotic Communication. The last category includes classic types of psychotic speech, as for example echolalia. This category developed from the early use of Pre-Therapy with psychotic populations. Researchers have either questioned its relevance (Brenner, 2006), or not used it at all. Prouty (1990) abandoned the procedure of a semi-structured interview for the PTRS-2 and instead observed clients' communication during Pre-Therapy sessions. Transcripts of sessions, sometimes annotated by the therapist or an observer, are divided in phrases – groups of words that grammatically function as a single unit. The PTRS-2 better captures the frequency of contact signs, as raters count incidences of contact signs in every phrase. For example, the phrase 'I am Jim' scores two on Reality, for both the pronoun 'I' and the name 'Jim' refer to a concrete person. Markers can also be syntactic; for example words and full sentences are markers of Social Communication. Raters also look for markers in therapist responses and transcript annotations, particularly for the Affect category. An emotion word produced by the client is a marker of Affect, but so is a remark made by the therapist about the client's facial expression, or an observer's comment about an emotionally significant gesture. Category scores have virtually no maximum. A PTRS-2 total score is generally not calculated.

Evaluation Criterion for the Pre-Therapy Interview

Dinacci (1997) found the PTRS-2 unsatisfactory for use with less verbal clients, as it relies heavily on verbal responses. He developed an alternative for evaluating contact functions in verbally disorganised clients, a rating scale for use with videotapes called the Evaluation Criterion for the Pre-Therapy Interview (ECPI). Although the ECPI can be used with the Pre-Therapy Interview, the level of verbal disorganisation in many clients precludes structured interview techniques (Dinacci, 1997; Lunardi, 2002). A scoring unit is defined as client behaviour immediately following a stimulus (e.g., a speaker turn) of the therapist or interviewer. Any *change* in the client's behaviour following a stimulus is considered a marker of contact. Change can be anything from a shift in posture to a verbal utterance, or even silence in a client who otherwise has not stopped talking. The assumption is that behaviour changes when it is affected by the stimulus. Scoring units demonstrative of change are termed *client responses*. The ECPI provides six indices of contact behaviour: (1) The Reaction Index is a measure of general client reactivity. It is the percentage of client responses relative to the total number of scoring units. (2) The Expressive Modality Index evaluates whether client responses are meaningfully related to the stimulus and the extent to which these responses are verbal. (3) The Verbal Expressiveness Index evaluates whether subsequent verbal responses are meaningfully interrelated. (4) The Coherence Index is calculated as the percentage of time that the client performed non-verbal behaviour in coordination with verbal behaviour. (5) The Physical Expressiveness Index measures the percentage of contact responses that involve touch, either as a stimulus from the therapist or a response from the client. (6) The General Interview Index (GII) is the mean of all previous indices. These indices have values between 0 and 100, with higher values indicative of more or more important markers of contact. Brenner (2006) has noted that the ECPI only accounts for client responses, not for client initiations of communication. She proposed additional measures of client contact behaviour that relate to Dinacci's Physical Expressiveness Index. She counted initiations of eye contact by the client, and registered duration of client initiated touch and eye contact.

Contact reflections

The English PTRS-2 contains brief instructions for the observation of therapist contact reflections, but these have never been used. Brenner (2006) developed her own guidelines for raters, while Schellevis (2006) let therapists categorise their own responses. Brenner also proposed that physical contact initiated by the therapist is relevant for Pre-Therapy and she has measured the duration of such events.

Conclusions

Both the PTRS-1 and 2 and the ECPI can be used to assess client contact behaviour during a semi-structured interview or a Pre-Therapy session. Interactions are registered so that raters can detect markers of contact in client behaviour. This typically requires painstaking, lengthy work (Strens, 2005; Van den Mooter, 2006). Scoring units vary from one complete reply or speaking turn within an interview (PTRS-1), to one grammatical unit (PTRS-2), to all client behaviour in a session (ECPI). The ECPI takes into account almost all non-verbal client behaviours, whereas the PTRS-2 takes into account only those with a clear affective connotation.

Reliability

Inter-rater reliability is the extent to which different raters agree when evaluating a scoring unit. Raters may not perfectly agree on the frequency of contact behaviour pertaining to one scoring unit, but perfectly agree that one scoring unit displays more contact behaviour relative to another.

Pre-Therapy Rating Scale

Brenner (2006) and Van den Mooter (2006) were both positive about the clarity of the PTRS-2 manual provided by De Vre (1992), but found that it lacked sufficient guidelines for the detection of non-verbal contact markers in the Affect category. We have calculated our own estimates of inter-rater agreement, based on the data set from Brenner (2006) and descriptive statistics reported in the literature.

Brenner (2006) and an independent rater applied the PTRS-2 on a ten-minute recording of a Pre-Therapy session with a 66-year-old male in-patient with mild intellectual disability. We calculated intraclass correlations between the raters (one-way random effect), based on the score for each category for every half minute. Agreement between the raters was low for Affect ($r = .07$), medium for Reality ($r = .48$) and high for Communication ($r = .81$). Clearly, PTRS-2 scores of one rater can differ greatly from the scores of another rater, particularly for the Affect scale. Alternatively, evidence for high inter-rater reliability can be drawn from Prouty's (1994, p. 46) report on a single session with a young woman with schizoaffective and intellectually limited processes. He reported PTRS-2 scores for the beginning, middle and end of that session (sampled at percentiles 1–20, 40–60, 80–100). We calculated an intraclass correlation for each of the categories and all correlations were almost perfect ($r > .96$). Intraclass correlations were also very high for each of the separately reported markers, including the non-verbal markers ($r > .96$). Visual inspection of the data reported by Prouty (1994, p. 46; Table 1) also suggests that raters can reach high levels of relative agreement when scores are calculated across multiple minutes. These observations suggest that Brenner's (2006) and Van den Mooter's (2006) suspicion of non-verbal markers in the PTRS-2 may not be totally warranted.

Three case studies have reported session scores from two to three raters, aggregated over months to obtain a session-independent estimate of contact (Table 2). Prouty (1990) reported on 100 Pre-Therapy sessions with a girl with intellectual disability, alternately diagnosed as schizophrenic, brain-damaged or autistic. Prouty and Cronwall (1990) have reported on the case of a depressed, non-verbal boy, with a Stanford-Binet IQ of 13. This client received 200 sessions from the same therapist over a period of two years. For both cases, PTRS-2 scores were reported per minute and averaged across all sessions in one year. Prouty (1994, p. 45) presents the treatment of a schizophrenic male with profound intellectual limitations. He reported means of category scores per session over three 3-month periods. Visual inspection of the data provided in these case studies suggests that raters within each study have reached high levels of agreement on all PTRS-2 categories (see Table 2). As raters within each study appear to have reached high levels of agreement on Affect, reported doubts about the detection of markers for the Affect scale may reflect differences between interpretations of the manual rather than difficulties in rating Affect reliably per se.

Evaluation Criterion for the Pre-Therapy Interview

Brenner (2006) and Van den Mooter (2006) were each independently unsatisfied with the vague definitions of *therapist stimuli* and *client responses* in the manual of the ECPI. Brenner (2006) has assessed ECPI reliability with a ten-minute recording of a Pre-Therapy session (see above). She reported moderate absolute agreement for the detection of client responses in scoring units ($k = .59$), which

Table 1

Contact response counts for PTRS-2 categories, with discrimination between clients, raters and phase of session

Study	Client	Phase	Rater	Reality	Affect	Social Communication
Prouty, 1994, p. 46	4	start	7	22	4	9
	4	start	8	24	3	12
	4	middle	7	105	12	57
	4	middle	8	96	13	53
	4	end	7	61	8	35
	4	end	8	51	8	25
Van den Mooter, 2006[a]	5	min. 1–5	9	5	3	8
	5	min. 6–10	9	0	1	0
	5	min. 11–15	9	2	5	2
	5	min. 16–20	9	4	3	3
	5	min. 21–25	9	3	2	3
	5	min. 26–30	9	8	1	8
	5	min. 31–35	9	6	2	4
	5	min. 36–40	9	0	0	0
	5	min. 41–45	9	4	3	5
	6	min. 1–5	9	0	12	0
	6	min. 6–10	9	0	13	0

[a] Response counts for clients 5 and 6 are calculated from the data set produced by Van den Mooter (2006)

is needed to calculate the Reaction Index. Absolute agreement was lower for the qualifications of client responses that are needed to calculate each of the remaining indices ($k < .36$). To test how well the raters agreed on the actual ECPI indices (range 0 to 100), we calculated intraclass correlations for each half-minute segment. We observed that raters agreed almost perfectly for the Physical Expressiveness Index ($r = .93$), and moderately for each of the other indices ($.35 < r < .65$). In all, preliminary findings of inter-rater reliability with the ECPI are promising, but the rating procedure needs improvement. In contrast to this, Brenner (2006) has established substantial reliability for registered occasions of eye contact and touch that were initiated by the client ($k = .80$).

Contact reflections

Brenner (2006) developed her own system to categorise contact reflections. Her system includes six categories: Situational Reflections, Word-for-Word Reflections, and verbal and non-verbal Facial and Body Reflections. She and an independent rater categorised the contact reflections in a 10-minute Pre-Therapy segment of a session with a 35-year-old female with mild intellectual disability and a pervasive developmental disorder. Brenner (2006) estimated inter-rater agreement as if the categories were mutually exclusive and the agreement was substantial (k = .78). However, these categories were actually not mutually exclusive. Therefore we have aggregated the data of Brenner (2006) into counts for half-minute segments and calculated intraclass correlations (one-way

Table 2

Average contact scores for PTRS-2 categories, with discrimination between clients, raters, and phase of treatment

Study	Client	Phase	Rater	Reality	Affect	Social Communication
Prouty, 1990[a]	1	year 1	1	1.05	0.22	1.33
	1	year 1	2	1.03	0.23	1.70
	1	year 2	1	6.46	1.13	3.52
	1	year 2	2	8.20	1.12	3.77
Prouty & Cronwall, 1990[b]	2	year 1	1	0.21	–	0.33
	2	year 1	3	0.22	–	0.37
	2	year 1	4	0.20	–	0.30
	2	year 2	1	1.18	–	1.82
	2	year 2	3	0.87	–	1.87
	2	year 2	4	1.15	–	1.78
Prouty, 1994, p. 45[b]	3	months 1–3	5	59.00	27.00	71.00
	3	months 1–3	6	48.00	27.00	77.00
	3	months 4–5	5	149.00	11.50	110.00
	3	months 4–5	6	175.00	11.50	100.00
	3	months 6–9	5	379.00	17.00	214.00
	3	months 6–9	6	446.00	13.00	225.00

[a] Number of contact responses per minute per session, averaged over one year
[b] Number of contact responses per session, averaged over three months

random effect). We observed high relative inter-rater agreement for each of the four verbal reflections ($r > .93$) but moderate to low agreement for the non-verbal body and facial reflections ($r = .76$; $r = .54$).

Conclusions

No reliability data was found concerning the PTRS-1. Some evidence of reliability for coding with the PTRS-2 and ECPI is emerging. For reliability of these measures to improve, the manuals of the PTRS-2 and particularly the ECPI are in need of elaboration. In particular, they should provide more information about the detection of non-verbal markers. Continuing evaluation of reliability should be part of any study that uses the ECPI or the PTRS. So far, researchers of contact behaviour have mainly assessed inter-rater reliability, but other types of reliability (test-retest, inter-item) should also be evaluated.

Construct validity

Construct validity refers to whether an instrument measures what it is supposed to measure. Reality contact and affective contact refer to the *awareness* of people/places/things and emotions respectively, while communicative contact has been defined consistently (Prouty, 1994; Prouty et al., 1998/2002) as the *symbolisation* of contact with reality and affect. The PTRS-1 and 2 and the ECPI are used to evaluate clients' communicative behaviour. As such, they are direct operationalisations of communicative contact, from which reality and affective contact are inferred. We have explored how the instruments under discussion relate to this construct. Where possible we have also examined whether the subscales within each instrument actually measure different constructs. We offer a similar discussion of the detection and categorisation of contact reflections.

Pre-Therapy Rating Scale

The authors of the PTRS-2 have consistently referred to its categories as contact dimensions (De Vre, 1992; Prouty, 1994; Prouty et al., 1998/2002), but dimensionality of the instrument has never been assessed. The similarity between contact functions and PTRS-2 categories can be misleading, as all categories primarily measure one function: communicative contact. The PTRS-2 does not reflect the three-function structure that is theorised by Prouty. In fact, there are two indications that the PTRS-2 measures two rather than three elements of contact. First, the Social Communication subscale is dependent on the Reality subscale. This is because both English (Prouty, 1990) and Dutch (De Vre, 1992) manuals state that contact responses in the Social Communication category should demonstrate at least one clear reference to reality. Second, the Affect category may confound measures of therapist or observer behaviour and client behaviour. This is because, unlike the verbal markers of the other categories, the non-verbal markers of Affect can be identified in therapist responses or observer notes.

To empirically assess the relation between contact response categories, we merged the data from four case studies (Prouty, 1990, 1994, p. 45, 1994, p. 46; Prouty & Cronwall, 1990) and then further extended this data set with contact response counts for five-minute segments from a data set provided by Van den Mooter (2006). Van den Mooter (2006) and Strens (2005) independently coded the two videotaped sessions described in Peters (1996) and Van Werde and Willemaers (1993). Based on these data, Van den Mooter constructed a definitive rating of the sessions. Our final merged data set is presented in Tables 1 and 2. Data cannot be compared across studies in absolute terms, because some values are absolute counts whereas others were averaged over a number of minutes or sessions. Therefore we first converted the data to standard distributed values, using the means and standard deviations within each study (Prouty, 1994, p. 45, 1994, p. 46; Van den Mooter, 2006) or across studies (Prouty, 1990; Prouty & Cronwall, 1990). A two-tailed test of the Pearson correlation between Reality and Social Communication suggests that these measures are highly associated (r = .94, n = 33, p < .001). On the other hand, Affect was not significantly associated with either category (r = .05, n = 27, n.s.; r = .05, n = 27, n.s.). These results offer preliminary support for a two-dimensional structure of the PTRS-2.

Evaluation Criterion for the Pre-Therapy Interview

Although developed for Pre-Therapy research, the ECPI does not clearly reflect Prouty's theory of the contact functions (Dinacci, 1997; Brenner, 2006). It includes no explicit evaluation of the symbolisation of reality or affective contact. Neither has the relation between its indices been evaluated. As this instrument primarily measures meaningfulness of communication, it is essentially a measure of language pragmatics. Pragmatic skills are defined as the ability to convey and understand intended meanings (Adams & Lloyd, 2005; Frith, 1993). They are distinguished from phonological, lexical and syntactic skills. Brenner (2006) has argued that communicative contact should not be limited to verbal behaviour, and Kelly (2001) has similarly argued that non-verbal exchanges of meaning are the basis of language pragmatics. The ability to engage in meaningful communication with others is traditionally studied in the field of developmental linguistics (e.g., Adams, 2001), but also in the context of schizophrenia (e.g., Linscott, 2005), autism (e.g., Eales, 1993), and gerontology (e.g., Intrieri & Morse, 1997).

Van den Mooter (2006) has recently evaluated the association of contact behaviour with language pragmatics using the PTRS-2, the ECPI and the Analysis of Language Impaired Children's Conversation (ALICC) (Bishop, Chan, Adams, Hartley & Weir, 2000). Two-step cluster analyses were conducted separately for verbal utterances (n = 75) and annotations of non-verbal behaviour (n = 597) observed in two videotaped Pre-Therapy sessions: one with a non-verbal female with profound intellectual limitations (Peters, 1996) and one with a verbal, schizophrenic female (Van Werde & Willemaers, 1993). The resulting clusters differentiated strongly between the cases, between subscales of the ALICC, and between various markers of contact. This finding supports the assumption that measures of contact are in fact measuring the ability to convey and understand meaning.

Contact reflections

Brenner (2006) categorised therapists' contact reflections in seven 10-minute segments of Pre-Therapy sessions with adults with intellectual disability. Brenner constructed contingency tables for the presence of client contact behaviour and therapist contact reflections in all five-second segments in her data set. She tested the likelihood of client contact behaviour co-occurring with therapist contact reflections using the j coefficient. Incidences of contact reflections and contact behaviour were contingent in all therapy sessions, supporting the assumption that therapist contact reflections and client contact behaviour are related.

Schellevis (2006) attempted to assess Prouty's typology of contact reflections using the videotaped sessions reported by Peters (1996) and Van Werde and Willemaers (1993). For this purpose she had the therapists categorise their own contact reflections. She further rated therapist interventions using the PTRS-2, the Hill Counselor Verbal Response Category System (HCVRCS) (Hill, 1986) and the ALICC. A two-step cluster analysis revealed two clusters that differentiated strongly between the cases, between various markers of contact, and between subscales of the HCVRCS and the ALICC. A two-step cluster analysis differentiated between various markers of contact and between subscales of the linguistic instruments, which again suggests that measures of contact are actually measuring the ability to convey and understand meaning. Additionally, these clusters differentiated between situational and word-for-word reflections, applied to a different extent in each case. This offers preliminary evidence for the validity of Prouty's (1976) typology of contact reflections, and it suggests that different types of contact reflection require different pragmatic skills.

Conclusions

In theory, the PTRS and the ECPI primarily measure communicative contact, but these instruments may actually assess the ability to convey and understand meaning. The PTRS-2 seems to measure two elements: one is dependent on client behaviour only, while the other is also dependent on therapist and/or observer behaviour. There is preliminary evidence that different contact reflections require different pragmatic skills.

Pre-Therapy process and outcome

We have aggregated the findings of all available publications on descriptive and comparative tests of Pre-Therapy. As far as we know there are no unpublished Pre-Therapy outcome studies (but we would be pleased to learn of others). *Descriptive* process-outcome evaluations assess whether communicative contact of Pre-Therapy clients improves over time and relates to client improvement. *Comparative* process-outcome evaluations assess whether communicative contact improves more in Pre-Therapy than in other treatments and also relates to improved outcomes.

Descriptive tests

Dinacci (1997) reports ECPI scores before and after treatment for two in-patients, both nearly mute and physically and/or intellectually disabled, diagnosed with schizophrenia and hospitalised for at least 30 years in the same psychiatric institution. They received Pre-Therapy twice a week during seven months, as well as a constant dose of neuroleptics before and during the observed period (Table 3). Treatment resulted in pre-post GII changes of 13 and 24 points ($t[1] =$ 3.36; n.s.; $d = .64$). These findings were associated with nursing observations of improvement (Dinacci, 1997).

Additional data on the relationship between increased communicative contact and outcome is available from three single-case studies (Prouty, 1990, 1994, p. 45; Prouty & Cronwall, 1990). All clients had multiple diagnoses, including schizophrenia or intellectual disability. Pre-Therapy treatment varied from nine months to two years, with up to 200 sessions. PTRS-2 data are presented in Table 2. Due to the fact that changes could not be directly compared across studies in absolute terms, the scores were first converted to standard distributed values and then averaged across raters. There was significant change in Social Communication from the beginning to the end of therapy ($t[2] = -8.88, p < .05, d = 2.17$). The sum of standard scores was calculated across all categories for each client and averaged over the raters to obtain a more general estimate of communicative contact. There was a large ($d = 1.44$) but not statistically significant change in communicative contact from the beginning to the end of therapy ($t[2] = 2.82$, n.s.).

We have used these findings to calculate an average, weighted effect size for improvement in contact process occurring as a result of Pre-Therapy treatment for schizophrenic patients. The total number of cases is very small ($n = 5$), but the result after nine to twenty-four months of treatment is large: $d = 1.08$ (95% CI between -.03 and 2.47). After treatment, the test score of an average person who received treatment was likely to be higher than 86% of similar patients before treatment. (Note that these small sample estimates are based on statistics that did not reach statistical significance.) Pre-Therapy does appear to improve the contact functioning of clients with schizophrenia in clinically significant ways.

Comparative test

Hinterkopf et al. (1979) conducted a randomised controlled study on a ward for chronic schizophrenic patients who had been hospitalised on average for 20 years. Seven pairs of in-patients were matched on pre-treatment PTRS-1 total scores and one client from each patient pair was randomly assigned to either the treatment or the control group. Seven participating therapists, all trained in client-centred/experiential psychotherapy and Pre-Therapy, offered one hour of individual attention per week to two patients, one of each treatment condition, for six months. The patients in the treatment group received Pre-Therapy during the allotted hour, whereas the patients in the control group received recreational therapy. On the basis of a post-treatment PTRS-1 evaluation, the number of patients with improved scores was counted for each of the categories. While the authors reported a higher number of improved patients for Communication of Basic Reality in the experimental group, this difference was not statistically significant (Fisher's exact test, $df = 1$, $p = .13$, Cohen's $d = .61$). Due to lack of information concerning the dimensional structure of the PTRS-1, we were unable to estimate the number of participants who had an improved score for at least one of the categories.

Finally, Dinacci (1997) compared the Pre-Therapy treatment of two in-patients with schizophrenia (reported above) to the regular treatment of two other in-patients from the same ward, matched for age, symptoms, GII score and duration of stay in the institution (Table 3). All of these patients received a constant dose of neuroleptics before and during the observed period. The difference in post-treatment GII scores for these pairs was not statistically

Table 3

ECPI pre- and post-General Interview Index (GII) for four schizophrenic inpatients, from Dinacci (1997)

Client	Gender	Age	Hospital-ization	Medication	Pre-Therapy	Pre-GII	Post-GII
A	male	45	30	propericiazine, diazepam	yes	18	42
B	male	67	55	propericiazine	yes	64	77
C	male	46	32	haloperidol	no	52	46
D	male	67	40	propericiazine	no	15	17

significant ($t[2]$ = 1.23; n.s.), even though the controlled effect size was large (d = .77). The size of these effects suggests that Pre-Therapy treatment could result in higher verbal expressivity and more meaningful communication, even in patients with schizophrenia who have over 30 years of hospitalisation.

With the studies by Hinterkopf et al. (1979) and Dinacci (1997) we can estimate an average, weighted effect size of Pre-Therapy in relation to an in-patient comparison group. This estimate is based on PTRS-1 Communication of Basic Reality and ECPI GII scores from 18 cases. The average effect size is large: d = .64 (95% CI between -.31 and 1.60). After six to seven months of Pre-Therapy treatment, the average in-patient with severe and chronic symptoms of schizophrenia can be expected to score higher on measures of contact behaviour than 74% of similar patients who did not receive this treatment.

Conclusions

Two small randomised controlled studies and three single-case studies have reported estimates of change in communicative contact in Pre-Therapy. All patients demonstrated chronic communicative and emotional problems relating to schizophrenia or intellectual disability. Average descriptive and controlled effect sizes for these studies are large, even though they lack statistical power. Still, with one of the more reliable subscales of the PTRS-2 (Social Communication) we found evidence from three single-case studies that communicative contact can improve over a period of one to two years. These clients produced more meaningful expressions in the last phase of treatment. However, we found no evaluation of the relation between improved communicative contact and other elements of client improvement, except for unsystematic reports by staff or family.

Discussion

Prouty (1976, 1990, 1994) distinguishes three functions of contact: reality contact, affective contact and communicative contact. Due to the manner of measurement of contact behaviour, Pre-Therapy researchers have consistently focused on the communicative function. They have screened clients' verbal and non-verbal expressions for markers of contact (Hinterkopf et al., 1979; Prouty, 1990; Dinacci, 1997; Brenner, 2006). Even though Prouty's theory of contact involves a shift from Rogers' interpersonal approach to a focus on contact within the individual, Pre-Therapy research has a strong interpersonal flavour because meaningfulness of communication is dependent on the context of communication and particularly the behaviour of others. We believe, therefore, that the theory and practice of Pre-Therapy could benefit from a clarification of its core concepts and processes by making use of tools from the field of language pragmatics. With its long tradition of accounting for referential and contextual aspects of communication, it offers the Pre-Therapy field a wealth of potential assessment tools and instruments (Adams, 2002). The developmental perspective of these instruments fits well with recent clarifications of Pre-Therapy theory and practice in terms of developmental psychology (Peters, 2005, 2006).

Contact reflections are supposed to meet the client at their level of expression and experiencing and to facilitate client contact efforts, hence supporting the formation of therapeutic and other relationships. Preliminary research findings generally support this view. Improvements in patients' PTRS or ECPI scores support the frequently reported subjective impressions of therapists, nursing staff and family. However, outcome research would benefit from studies with more reliable measures and larger treatment groups. Evaluations of training as performed by Ondracek (2004) can also be used in valuable tests of outcome. More frequent single-case studies (see Elliott, 2002) will also be useful in evaluating the efficacy of Pre-Therapy. The only statistically significant outcome effect in our review was obtained by aggregating three single-case studies. Studies focusing on in-session client change in relation to therapist goals and interventions could help practitioners develop a task model for Pre-Therapy (see Greenberg, 1984). Such a model would help researchers to compare case reports and support future and larger outcome studies.

Finally, we encourage a broad range of practitioners to publish process and outcome findings on Pre-Therapy in particular and contact functions in general. Contact reflections are currently applied in psychotherapy, special education, and nursing, and not only for people with schizophrenia. Systematic research, including single-case studies, on all populations and all types of practitioners is required to advance the field of Pre-Therapy.

References

Adams, C (2001) Clinical diagnostic and intervention studies of children with semantic-pragmatic language disorder. *International Journal of Language and Communication Disorders, 36,* 289–305.

Adams, C (2002) Practitioner review: The assessment of language pragmatics. *Journal of Child Psychology and Psychiatry, 43,* 973–87.

Adams, C & Lloyd, J (2005) Elicited and spontaneous communicative functions and stability of conversational measures with children who have pragmatic language impairments. *International Journal of Language and Communication Disorders, 40,* 333–47.

Beadle-Brown, JD & Whiten, A (2004) Elicited imitation in children and adults with autism: Is there a deficit? *Journal of Intellectual & Developmental Disability, 29,* 147–63.

Bishop, DVM, Chan, J, Adams, C, Hartley, J & Weir, F (2000) Conversational responsiveness in specific language impairment: Evidence of disproportionate pragmatic difficulties in a subset of children with specific language impairment. *Development and Psychopathology, 12,* 177–99.

Brenner, N (2006) *Auf der Suche nach Kontakt. Analyse der Prä-Therapie nach Garry F. Prouty bei Menschen mit einer geistigen Behinderung und Kontaktstörungen.* Unpublished master's thesis, Universität Koblenz-Landau, Landau.

Buber, M (1964) Phenomenological analysis of existence versus pointing to the concrete (M Friedman et al, Trans). In M Friedman (Ed) *The Worlds of Existentialism: A critical reader* (pp. 547–9). New York: Random House. (Reprinted from *Eclipse of God. Studies in the relation between religion and philosophy* by M Buber, 1957, New York: Harper Torchbooks.)

De Vre, R (1992) *Prouty's Pre-Therapie.* Unpublished master's thesis. Rijksuniversiteit Gent, Faculteit Psychologie en Pedagogische Wetenschappen, Gent, Belgium.

Dinacci, A (1997) Ricerca sperimentale sul trattamento psicologico dei pazienti schizophrenici con la pre-therapia di Dr G Prouty. *Psicologia della Persona, 2,* 32–49.

Dodds, P, Morton, I & Prouty, G (2004) Using Pre-Therapy techniques in dementia care. *Journal of Dementia Care, 12,* 25–8.

Eales, MJ (1993) Pragmatic impairments in adults with childhood diagnoses of autism or developmental receptive language disorder. *Journal of Autism and Developmental Disorders, 23,* 593–617.

Elliott, R (2002) Hermeneutic single-case efficacy design. *Psychotherapy Research, 12,* 1–21.

Fonagy, P, Gergely, G, Jurist, EL & Target, M (Eds) (2002) *Affect Regulation, Mentalization and the Development of the Self.* New York: Other Press.

Frith, CD (1993) *The Cognitive Neuropsychology of Schizophrenia.* Hove: Erlbaum.

Greenberg, LS (1984) Task analysis: The general approach. In LN Rice & LS Greenberg (Eds) *Patterns of Change: Intensive analysis of psychotherapy process* (pp. 124–48). New York: Guilford.

Hill, CE (1986) An overview of the Hill counselor and client verbal response modes category systems. In LS Greenberg & WM Pinsof (Eds) *The Psychotherapeutic Process: A research handbook* (pp. 131–60). New York: Guilford.

Hill, CE & Lambert, MJ (2003) Methodological issues in studying psychotherapy processes and outcomes. In MJ Lambert (Ed) *Handbook of Psychotherapy and Behavior Change* (5th ed) (pp. 84–136). New York: Wiley.

Hinterkopf, E, Prouty, G & Brunswick, L (1979) A pilot study of Pre-Therapy method applied to chronic schizophrenic patients. *Psychosocial Rehabilitation Journal, 3,* 11–19.

Intrieri, RC & Morse, JM (1997) A sequential analysis of verbal and nonverbal interaction of two long-term care residents. *Journal of Applied Gerontology, 16,* 477–94.

Kelly, SD (2001) Broadening the units of analysis in communication: Speech and nonverbal behaviours in pragmatic comprehension. *Journal of Child Language, 28,* 325–49.

Linscott, RJ (2005) Thought disorder, pragmatic language impairment, and generalized cognitive decline in schizophrenia. *Schizophrenia Research, 75,* 225–32.

Lunardi, C (2002) Pre-Therapy treatment with employment of Evaluation Criterion of Pre-Therapy Interview (ECPI): A case. *Pre-Therapy International Review, 2,* 25–7.

Ondracek, P (2004) Personzentriertes Arbeiten und Kontaktförderung. Ansatz zur Wirksamkeitserfassung. In H Greving (Ed) *Jahrbuch Heilpädagogik 2004. Aktuelle Entwicklungen und Tendenzen in der Heilpädagogik* (pp. 75–124). Berlin: BHP-Verlag.

Peters, H (1996) Toepassing van Prouty's pretherapeutische methoden in de behandeling van geestelijk gehandicapten. *Tijdschrift voor Orthopedagogiek, Kinderpsychiatrie en klinische Kinderpsychologie, 21,* 23–36.

Peters, H (1999) Pre-Therapy: A client-centered/experiential approach to mentally handicapped people. *Journal of Humanistic Psychology, 39,* 8–29.

Peters, H (2005) Pre-Therapy from a developmental perspective. *Journal of Humanistic Psychology, 45*, 62–81.

Peters, H (2006) The development of intersubjectivity in relation to psychotherapy and its importance for Pre-Therapy. *Person-Centered & Experiential Psychotherapies, 5*, 191–207.

Pörtner, M (2000) *Trust and Understanding: The person-centred approach to everyday care for people with special needs.* Ross-on-Wye: PCCS Books. (Original work published 1996)

Prouty, G (1976) Pre-Therapy – A method of treating pre-expressive psychotic and retarded patients. *Psychotherapy: Theory, Research and Practice, 13*, 290–5.

Prouty, G (1990) A theoretical evolution in the person-centered/experiential psychotherapy of schizophrenia and retardation. In G Lietaer, J Rombauts & R Van Balen (Eds) *Client-Centered and Experiential Psychotherapy in the Nineties* (pp. 645–85). Leuven, Belgium: Leuven University Press.

Prouty, G (1994) *Theoretical Evolutions in Person-Centered/Experiential Therapy. Applications to schizophrenic and retarded psychoses.* New York: Praeger.

Prouty, G & Cronwall M (1990). Psychotherapy with a depressed mentally retarded adult: An application of Pre-Therapy. In A Dosen & F Menolascino (Eds) *Depression in Mentally Retarded Children and Adults* (pp. 281–93). Leiden: Logon Publicaties.

Prouty, G, Van Werde, D & Pörtner, M (2002) *Pre-Therapy: Reaching contact-impaired clients.* Ross-on-Wye: PCCS Books. (Original work published 1998)

Rogers, CR (1957) The necessary and sufficient conditions of therapeutic personality change. *Journal of Consulting Psychology, 21*, 95–103.

Sanders, P & Wyatt, G (2002) The history of conditions one and six. In G Wyatt & P Sanders (Eds) *Rogers' Therapeutic Conditions: Evolution, theory and practice. Vol 4: Contact and Perception* (pp. 1–24). Ross-on-Wye: PCCS Books.

Schellevis, A (2006) *A psycholinguistic analysis of the contact reflection.* Unpublished master's thesis. Katholieke Universiteit Leuven, Faculteit Psychologie en Pedagogische Wetenschappen, Leuven, Belgium.

Strens, J (2005) *La Pré-Therapie développée par Prouty: Un concept théorique et practique au sein de l'Approche Centrée sur la Personne.* Unpublished master's thesis. Université Catholique de Louvain, Faculté Sciences Psychologiques, Louvain-La-Neuve, Belgium.

Van den Mooter, B (2006) *Een psycholinguïstische analyse van contactgedrag.* Unpublished master's thesis. Katholieke Universiteit Leuven, Faculteit Psychologie en Pedagogische Wetenschappen, Leuven, Belgium.

Van Werde, D & Morton, I (1999) The relevance of Prouty's Pre-Therapy to dementia care. In I Morton (Ed) *Person-Centred Approaches to Dementia Care* (pp. 139–66). Bicester: Winslow Press.

Van Werde, D & Willemaers, R (1993) *Werken aan Contact: Een illustratie van Pre-Therapie met een chronisch psychotische vrouw.* Rijksuniversiteit Gent, Faculteit van de Psychologische en Pedagogische Wetenschappen, Gent, Belgium.

Wyatt, G & Sanders, P (Eds) (2002) *Rogers' Therapeutic Conditions: Evolution, theory and practice. Vol 4: Contact and Perception.* Ross-on-Wye: PCCS Books.

Contributors

Editors

Peter Pearce is Head of the Person-Centred Department at Metanoia Institute, UK where, amongst other trainings, he runs an MSc in Contemporary Person-Centred Psychotherapy, BA in Counselling, and the Practitioner Certificate in Person-Centred Practice at the Difficult Edge. He has provided person-centred counselling for nearly 25 years, predominantly in 'difficult edge' situations within the UK's National Health Service, multi-disciplinary community teams for adults with mental health issues and adults with learning disabilities, and with young people in Inner London school settings.

Lisbeth Sommerbeck is a clinical psychologist accredited as a specialist in psychotherapy by the Danish Psychological Association. She has worked in psychiatric settings for 35 years and is now retired. She is a member of the Pre-Therapy International Network and the founder of the recently created Danish Carl Rogers Forum. She has written many journal articles and two books, including *The Client-Centred Therapist in Psychiatric Contexts: A therapist's guide to the psychiatric landscape and its inhabitants* (PCCS Books, 2003).

Contributors

Pamela Bruce-Hay trained in person-centred counselling and has worked with people with dementia and families. She has used Pre-Therapy contact work in practice.

Mathias Dekeyser works as a psychologist for a clinical outreach service in Leuven, Belgium. He has worked as a researcher at the Center for Client-Centered/Experiential Psychotherapy and Counseling at the Catholic University of Leuven. He is currently working on a doctoral dissertation about body-oriented interventions.

Penny Dodds is a nurse with Sussex Partnership NHS Foundation Trust (mental health) and a lecturer at the University of Brighton. Having worked with people with dementia and older persons' mental health for a number of years, she has a specialist interest in working with people where communication and connections are challenging for staff.

Robert Elliott, PhD, is Professor of Counselling at the University of Strathclyde, and Professor Emeritus of Psychology at the University of Toledo. He has served as co-editor of the journals *Psychotherapy Research* and *Person-Centered & Experiential Psychotherapies*. He is co-author of three books, including *Learning Emotion-Focused Therapy: The process-experiential approach to change* and *Research Methods in Clinical Psychology: An introduction for students and practitioners* (Wiley, 2002), as well as more than 150 journal articles and book chapters. In 2008 he received the Distinguished Research Career Award from the Society for Psychotherapy Research and the Carl Rogers Award from the Division of Humanistic Psychology of the American Psychological Association.

Jan Hawkins is a person-centred practitioner, supervisor and freelance trainer. In 1994 Jan created, and co-facilitated, a diploma course in Counselling Survivors of Childhood Abuse, which ran for several years; the first initiative of its kind in Europe. Jan is committed to working with clients who have the widest range of abilities (including severe learning disabilities) in her practice. She has continued to run post-counselling training courses with a conviction that experiential learning is imperative for developing empathy as well as skills (www.janhawkins.co.uk).

Stephen Joseph, PhD, is Professor of Psychology at the University of Nottingham, UK. He received his MSc in social psychology from the London School of Economics and his PhD from the Institute of Psychiatry in London. His research is on positive psychology, psychotherapy and psychological trauma. Joseph's latest book, *What Doesn't Kill Us* was released in paperback in 2013 (Piatkus).

Danuta Lipinska, MA, author of *Person-Centred Counselling for People with Dementia: Making sense of self* (Jessica Kingsley, 2009), pioneered counselling persons with dementia. Her master's degree in counselling is from the University of New Hampshire, USA. Danuta developed training programmes in the United States and UK. She developed specialist counselling services for people with dementia and their relatives in London in the 1990s. Currently she is a tutor on the post-graduate diploma in person-centred counselling at the Norwich Centre for Counselling, Associate Dementia Specialist at the University of Worcester, and Action Learning Facilitator of the 'My Home Life: Leadership Support Programme' at City University, London.

David Murphy, PhD, is the programme leader for the MA in Person-Centred Experiential Counselling and Psychotherapy at the University of Nottingham, UK. He is a person-centred psychotherapist and Honorary Psychologist in Psychotherapy at the Centre for Trauma, Resilience and Growth, Nottinghamshire Healthcare NHS Trust. David has co-edited two books: *Relational Depth: New perspective and developments* (Palgrave MacMillan, 2012) and *Trauma and the Therapeutic Relationship: Approaches to process and practice* (Palgrave MacMillan, 2013). In addition to publishing numerous journal articles in the field of person-centered psychotherapy he is currently editor for the international journal *Person-Centered & Experiential Psychotherapies.*

Hans Peters is a registered healthcare psychologist. He is a supervisor of the Flemish Association of Client-Centered Therapy. He worked in an institution for the care of people with learning disabilities for 32 years, until his retirement in 1999. He has published more than 50 titles. For 13 years he was a member of the editorial board of the Dutch *Journal of Client-centered Psychotherapy.*

Garry Prouty (1936–2009) was trained by Eugene Gendlin at the University of Chicago. He developed his own therapeutic approach, Pre-Therapy, at clinics and hospitals for people with psychosis and severe learning disabilities. He lectured on Pre-Therapy in European clinics, hospitals and training organisations for over 17 years. Garry Prouty was founder of the Pre-Therapy International Network, a Fellow of the Chicago Counseling Center, and honorary member of the Chicago Psychological Association. He published widely in journals world-wide, and his books include *Theoretical Evolutions in Person-Centered/Experiential Therapy: Applications to schizophrenic and retarded psychoses* (Praeger, 1994), *Pre-Therapy: Reaching contact-impaired clients* (PCCS Books, 2002) and *Emerging Developments in Pre-Therapy* (PCCS Books, 2008).

Anja Rutten is a part-time senior lecturer in Autism at Sheffield Hallam University's Autism Centre, UK. She also has a private therapy, supervision, training and consultancy practice in Nottingham, where she works with a wide range of clients, with and without autism. Until recently, Anja was Head of Counselling and Research for Midlands Psychology, a Community Interest Company. Before that, she worked as a senior lecturer in Counselling and Psychotherapy at Staffordshire University and as Head of Social Programmes and Befriending for the National Autistic Society. Anja has a first degree in Psychology and an MA in Counselling and Psychotherapy and is currently studying for a PhD in Counselling Psychology. Anja's first training was in the person-centred approach, with additional training in emotion-focused therapy and Pre-Therapy. Her current research interests focus on how people with autism experience therapy.

Ros Sewell has provided person-centred counselling with young people within NHS and education settings since 1989. Ros is a primary tutor for the Post Qualification Conversion Diploma from Adult to Adolescent and School Counselling at Metanoia Institute and until recently was Competence Frameworks Manager for the British Association for Counselling and Psychotherapy (BACP). Ros is undertaking doctoral research on counselling in schools and has written and presented widely on these topics. She is currently joint Principal Investigator (with Peter Pearce) for the Align Project: An efficacy study of school-based counselling and was part of the BACP expert reference group for development of a Competence Framework for Counselling with Children and Young People.

Sally Stapleton is a chartered clinical psychologist working with people with dementia, their families, carers and staff teams in Sussex Partnership NHS Foundation Trust. Sally is a licensed Dementia Care Mapping Trainer with the Bradford Dementia Group (University of Bradford). She is particularly committed to promoting person-centred care within organisations.

Wendy Traynor is a senior lecturer at Liverpool John Moores University where she teaches on both the research-based MA in Counselling and Psychotherapeutic Practice and the post-graduate diploma in Counselling and Psychotherapy. She also worked for over 20 years in mental health services across all sectors in various roles including as therapist and supervisor, working with adults, children, young people and families.

Margaret Warner, PhD, is a Professor and Clinical Psychology faculty member at the Illinois School of Professional Psychology at Argosy University, Chicago. She is a client-centred therapist with a broad interest in empathic, relational styles of psychotherapy. She did her clinical training at the Chicago Counseling and Psychotherapy Center, an offshoot of the original centre founded by Carl Rogers. Margaret Warner has particular interest in humanistic therapy with severely disturbed clients, in family systems, and in multicultural groups. She has been a practising psychotherapist for over 20 years and has been teaching in client-centred therapy and psychopathology since 1983. She has published widely and has offered many presentations to international groups and conferences. She is a founding member of the World Association for Person-Centered and Experiential Psychotherapy and Counseling.

Dion Van Werde is a clinical psychologist, with a postgraduate specialisation in client-centred and experiential psychotherapy from Leuven University, Belgium. He is a founding member, with Jill and Garry Prouty, and coordinator and trainer, of the Pre-Therapy International Network. Dion is a co-author of *Pre-Therapy: Reaching contact-impaired clients* (PCCS Books, 2002). He works as a ward psychologist in Psychiatrisch Ziekenhuis Sint-Camillus in Gent, Belgium, where he uses Pre-Therapy to create a contact-ward milieu. He is an editorial board member of *Person-Centered & Experiential Psychotherapies*.

Index